AGITATION IN PATIENTS WITH DEMENTIA

A Practical Guide to Diagnosis and Management

Edited by

Donald P. Hay, M.D.

David T. Klein, Psy.D.

Linda K. Hay, R.N., Ph.D.

George T. Grossberg, M.D.

John S. Kennedy, M.D., F.R.C.P.C.

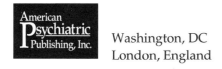

Washington, DC
London, England

Copyright © 2003 American Psychiatric Publishing, Inc.
ALL RIGHTS RESERVED

Manufactured in the United States of America on acid-free paper
07 06 05 04 03   5 4 3 2 1
First Edition

Because of their affiliation with Eli Lilly and Company, Drs. Donald and Linda Hay did not participate in the editorial review of those portions of this book discussing Lilly products.

Typeset in Adobe's Palatino and Futura

American Psychiatric Publishing, Inc.
1400 K Street, N.W.
Washington, DC 20005
www.appi.org

Library of Congress Cataloging-in-Publication Data
Agitation in patients with dementia : a practical guide to diagnosis and
    management / edited by Donald P. Hay ... [et al.].
        p. ; cm. -- (Clinical practice series)
    Includes bibliographical references and index.
    ISBN 0-88048-843-3 (alk. paper)
    1. Dementia--Complications. 2. Agitation (Psychology) I. Hay, Donald P.
II. Clinical practice (Unnumbered)
    [DNLM: 1. Dementia--complications. 2. Psychomotor Agitation--etiology.
WM 220 A2676 2002]
RC521 .A365 2002
616.8'3--dc21

                                                                2001045811

British Library Cataloguing in Publication Data
A CIP record is available from the British Library.

Contents

Contributors

Karin Barkin, M.D.
Instructor, Psychiatry and Behavioral Science, Medical University of South Carolina, Charleston

Daryl L. Bohac, Ph.D
Assistant Professor, Department of Psychiatry, University of Nebraska Medical Center, Omaha, Nebraska

Deanna Chesley, Pharm.D.
Clinical Pharmacy Coordinator, St. Mary's Health Center, St. Louis, Missouri

Jiska Cohen-Mansfield, Ph.D.
Director, Research Institute on Aging of the Hebrew Home of Greater Washington, Rockville, Maryland; Professor, Department of Health Care Sciences and School of Public Health, George Washington University, Washington, D.C.

Elizabeth Cookson, M.D.
Assistant Professor of Psychiatry, University of Colorado School of Medicine; Medical Director, Inpatient Behavioral Health, Denver Health Medical Center, Denver, Colorado

Susan Eller, M.A., R.N.
Saint Louis University Hospital, Department of Nursing, St. Louis, Missouri

David G. Folks, M.D.
Professor and Chair, Department of Psychiatry, University of Nebraska Medical Center, Omaha, Nebraska

Kari L. Franson, Pharm.D.
Associate Professor, College of Pharmacy, Western University of Health Sciences; Adjunct Associate Professor, Department of Psychiatry, Saint Louis University School of Medicine, St. Louis, Missouri

Barbara J. Gilchrist, J.D., Ph.D.
Saint Louis University School of Law, St. Louis, Missouri

Linda Griffin, R.N.C.
Saint Louis University Hospital, Department of Nursing, St. Louis, Missouri

George T. Grossberg, M.D.
Professor and Director of Geriatric Psychiatry, Department of Psychiatry and Human Behavior, Saint Louis University School of Medicine, St. Louis, Missouri

David Harper, Ph.D.
Assistant Director for Research, Geriatric Psychiatry Program, McLean Hospital, Belmont, Massachusetts; Instructor in Psychology, Department of Psychiatry, Harvard Medical School, Boston, Massachusetts

Linda K. Hay, Ph.D.[*]
Medical Liaison, Eli Lilly and Company, Indianapolis, Indiana; Adjunct Assistant Clinical Professor, Saint Louis University School of Medicine, St. Louis, Missouri

Donald P. Hay, M.D.
Clinical Research Physician, Eli Lilly and Company, Indianapolis, Indiana; Adjunct Clinical Associate Professor of Psychiatry, Department of Psychiatry, Saint Louis University, St. Louis, Missouri

John S. Kennedy, M.D., F.R.C.P.C.
Professor of Geriatric Psychiatry, Department of Psychiatry, Indiana University School of Medicine, Indianapolis, Indiana

David T. Klein, Psy.D.
St. Louis Veterans Administration Medical Center; Department of Psychiatry, Saint Louis University, St. Louis, Missouri

Leeanne Lott, M.S.W., L.C.S.W.
Division of Geriatric Psychiatry, Department of Psychiatry, Saint Louis University, St. Louis, Missouri

---

[*]Deceased

Rebekah Loy, Ph.D.
Research Associate Professor of Neurology, University of Rochester Medical Center, Program in Neurobehavioral Therapeutics, Monroe Community Hospital, Rochester, New York

Dennis P. McNeilly, Psy.D
Assistant Professor, Department of Psychiatry, University of Nebraska Medical Center, Omaha, Nebraska

Jacobo E. Mintzer, M.D.
Professor of Psychiatry, Psychiatry and Behavioral Science, Medical University of South Carolina, Charleston

Christine Mote, M.S.N., R.N.C.S.
Department of Nursing, Saint Louis University Hospital, St. Louis, Missouri

Anton Porsteinsson, M.D.
Assistant Professor of Psychiatry, University of Rochester Medical Center, Program in Neurobehavioral Therapeutics, Monroe Community Hospital, Rochester, New York

Yvette Rheaume, R.N.
Case Manager, E. N. Rogers Memorial Veterans Hospital, Bedford, Massachusetts

Mercedes M. Rodriguez, M.D.
Assistant Clinical Professor, Department of Psychiatry, Saint Louis University School of Medicine, St. Louis, Missouri; Staff Psychiatrist, Oarland Park OPC, Oarland Park, Florida

Andrew Satlin, M.D.
Director, Neuroscience Therapeutic Area, Novartis Pharmaceuticals Corporation, East Hanover, New Jersey; Research Associate in Psychiatry, Department of Psychiatry, Harvard Medical School, Boston, Massachusetts

Pierre N. Tariot, M.D.
Professor of Psychiatry, Medicine, and Neurology, University of Rochester Medical Center, Program in Neurobehavioral Therapeutics, Monroe Community Hospital, Rochester, New York

Ladislav Volicer, M.D., Ph.D.
Professor of Pharmacology and Psychiatry, Boston University School of Medicine, Boston, Massachusetts; Clinical Director, GRECC, E. N. Rogers Memorial Veterans Hospital, Bedford, Massachusetts

Joy Webster, M.D., M.P.H.
Assistant Clinical Professor, Department of Psychiatry and Human Behavior, Saint Louis University School of Medicine, St. Louis, Missouri

Steven P. Wengel, M.D.
Associate Professor, Department of Psychiatry, University of Nebraska Medical Center, Omaha, Nebraska

Perla Werner, Ph.D.
Department of Gerontology, Faculty of Social Welfare and Health Studies, University of Haifa, Haifa, Israel

Introduction
to the Clinical Practice Series

The Clinical Practice Series is dedicated to the support of continuing education and enrichment for the practicing clinician. Books in this series address topics of concern and importance to psychiatrists and other mental health clinicians. Each volume provides up-to-date literature reviews and emphasizes the most recent treatment approaches to psychiatric illnesses. Theoretical and scientific data are applied to clinical situations, and case illustrations are used extensively to increase the relevance of the material for the practitioner.

Each year the series publishes a number of books dealing with all aspects of clinical practice. From time to time, some of these publications may be revised and updated. Some books in the series are written by a single clinician widely acknowledged to be an authority on the topic area; other series books are edited volumes in which knowledgeable practitioners contribute chapters in their areas of expertise. Still other series books have their origins in presentations for an American Psychiatric Association Annual Meeting. All contain the newest research and clinical information available on the subjects discussed.

The Clinical Practice Series provides enrichment reading in a compact format specially designed to meet the continuing-education needs of the busy mental health clinician.

Judith H. Gold, C.M., M.D., F.R.C.P.C., F.R.A.N.Z.C.P.
Series Editor

Introduction

Donald P. Hay, M.D.

The number of individuals over the age of 65 years is rapidly increasing in this country, and the most rapidly rising segment of our population is adults age 85 years and older. Obviously, this aging-population explosion has far-reaching effects related not only to our personal experience but also to our professional roles as health care providers.

As knowledge about aging grows, myths and traditional thought give way to acceptance of new ways of thinking about getting older. No longer is the word *senility* politically correct, because this word is pejorative in its very essence, implying that just to be old means to be infirm. Disturbances in affect (depression), behavior (agitation), and cognition (dementia)—the "ABCs" of geriatric psychiatry—are not a part of normal aging. *Senile dementia* is an incorrect term because dementia is pathology and is not normal at any age.

This monograph, *Agitation in Patients with Dementia*, focuses on the "B" of the ABCs of geriatric psychiatry—that is, the agitation and behavioral disorders that are so obviously distressing for the individuals themselves, their families, the immediate professional caregivers, and the professional consultants. Health care professionals called on to help relieve the distress of an agitated patient with dementia face many challenges: identifying and diagnosing the multiple types of agitation in patients with dementia, looking for and treating the underlying medical etiologies, and recommending treatment and management techniques. This process can be overwhelming not only for the afflicted individuals but also for everyone charged with their care, including family and professional caregivers.

As a geriatric psychiatrist, I have often been called in the middle of the night by nursing home staff who are in urgent need of a solution for a patient who is not only obviously in distress but also disturbing other patients and staff. Such a call is the hallmark of this compelling treatment issue. This situation is often the most frustrating and challenging for health care professionals. We often wish that we had a magic pill or a sure-fire technique to recommend, but unfortunately we do not.

It is for this reason that we have undertaken the project of compiling this monograph from contributions of national and international experts in the field of diagnosing and treating agitation in patients with dementia.

Increasing attention has been focused on diagnosis and treatment of the agitation experienced by patients with dementia, and the literature in this area has grown correspondingly. This monograph is intended to serve as a comprehensive practical guide for the reader to help in integrating existing information and thereby to assist in the assessment and treatment of geriatric patients with dementia. The chapters have been written by experts—nationally and internationally respected leaders—in this field. Every contributor has had experience assessing patients and recommending and/or initiating treatments to alleviate agitation in these patients. The audience for this monograph includes geriatric psychiatrists, geriatricians, primary care physicians, internists, general practitioners, nurses, social workers, psychologists, pharmacists, mental health workers, and mental health practitioners—anyone working in hospitals, nursing homes, mental health centers and clinics, geriatric clinics, and pharmacies.

The subjects of the chapters in this book describe the field: agitation in the elderly: definitional and theoretical conceptualizations; epidemiology of agitation; neurochemistry of agitation; use of behavioral assessment scales for evaluating agitation in dementia; differential diagnosis of agitation in dementia: psychiatric conditions—delirium, depression, psychosis, and anxiety; clinical assessment and management of agitation in residential settings; nursing care adaptations, behavioral interventions, environmental changes, and sensory enhancement: conceptual, process, and outcome issues; psychotherapeutic interventions; bright light therapy; serotonergic agents; mood stabilizers; antipsychotic agents; beta-blockers, benzodiazepines, and other miscellaneous agents; electroconvulsive therapy; hormone therapies; and legal and ethical issues.

The authors and the editors of this monograph hope that you derive as much assistance from this effort as we have.

Dedication in Memoriam

Linda K. Hay, R.N., Ph.D.

This book is dedicated in memory of Linda Hay. Linda was a very special individual who foresaw the need for a text dealing with the most common of behavioral disturbances in psychogeriatrics: agitation. It was Linda's vision and leadership that brought together the many outstanding contributors to this volume.

Linda Hay was a remarkable person; a wife, mother, nurse, and geropsychologist. She attained national recognition in the field of geriatric psychiatry as a clinician and educator. Linda also established one of the first and largest Clinical Trial Units in Geriatric Psychiatry at Saint Louis University. Toward the end of her much too short life, she joined Eli Lilly & Company and began to establish a national network of geriatric psychiatrists.

Linda Hay was known as a doer. A person of action. Someone who took on both personal and professional challenges with gusto. No challenge was too great for Linda. She always approached adversity with a positive, can-do attitude. Those who came into contact with Linda were also impressed by her intellect, energy level, warm personality, and sense of humor. She is dearly missed by her family, friends, and colleagues, and by the field of Geriatric Psychiatry.

The Editors

I am grateful to the other editors for dedicating this book to the memory of my beloved wife. Linda's memory lives on as an inspiration to all. We miss her dearly, but her spirit and wisdom will be with us forever.

Donald P. Hay, M.D.

CHAPTER 1

Agitation in the Elderly

Definitional and Theoretical Conceptualizations

Jiska Cohen-Mansfield, Ph.D.

Inappropriate behaviors, or *agitation,* in the elderly are of great concern. These behaviors have a direct impact on the elderly person's caregivers as well as a direct and indirect impact on the elderly person him- or herself. Moreover, these behaviors may also indicate the person's internal experiences. Although there is universal consensus about the importance of these behaviors, controversies exist around many of the issues related to problem behaviors, including the domains included in and the etiology of these behaviors. In this chapter, these issues are described in detail.

Domains Included in Problem Behaviors

Agitation has been defined as "inappropriate verbal, vocal, or motor activity that is not judged by an outside observer to result directly from the needs or confusion of the individual" (Cohen-Mansfield and Billig 1986). Defining problem behaviors in this way results in an approach that includes the following attributes:

- **There is a range of behaviors.** Problem behaviors include repetitive acts (e.g., walking back and forth or repetition of words); behaviors inappropriate to the social norms (e.g., going into someone else's room and handling their belongings or unbuttoning a blouse in public); and aggressive behaviors toward the self or others. These behaviors have been labeled *problem behaviors, disruptive behaviors, disturbing behaviors, behavioral problems,* and *agitation;* all of these terms are generally used interchangeably.

- **Behavior is in the eye of the beholder.** In other words, problem behaviors are labeled as such by those who perceive them as inappropriate. However, a given behavior may or may not be inappropriate from the point of view of the older person. He or she may, indeed, have a need that explains the behavior but is not obvious to the observer. Furthermore, this need may not be consciously known by the older person. For example, a person who is walking incessantly may be searching for the bathroom; not only does he or she not make this need known to others, but he or she also may not be consciously aware of this need because of dementia.

- **The behaviors are not necessarily disruptive.** It is important to observe these behaviors because they may reveal the internal state of the older person. Repetitious mannerisms, although not bothersome to anyone, may indicate boredom; low groans that are not disruptive may nevertheless indicate pain.

- **The person does not necessarily suffer from dementia.** Although problem behaviors are more common among those suffering from dementia, some of these behaviors are also manifested by persons who are not cognitively impaired (Koss et al. 1997).

- **The behaviors are not necessarily outcomes of dementia.** The term *problem behaviors* does not refer to behaviors associated with dementia-related deterioration, such as memory problems or incontinence in the later stages of disease. Although many elderly people with dementia manifest problem behaviors, not all do.

- **The behaviors are observable behaviors with no underlying emotional state.** The problem behavior is an observable behavior, and no underlying emotional state is assumed to cause the behavior. In this sense, the label *agitation* is deceptive. It was only chosen because it has traditionally been used by practitioners to describe these behaviors.

Topics of Controversy

Different researchers have examined different domains and populations when studying agitation. Some investigators have included only persons with dementia, and others have considered only behaviors that were disruptive to others. Most importantly, some researchers have grouped other clusters of behaviors under this category, including memory problems, problems in the performance of activities of daily living, delusions, hallucinations, sleep problems, and depression. This combining of behaviors is evident in assessment instruments that include some or all of these problems. For example, the Behavioral Pathology in Alzheimer's Disease Rating Scale (BEHAVE-AD; Reisberg et al. 1987) assesses paranoid or delusional ideation, hallucinations, diurnal rhythm disturbance, affective disturbance, and anxieties and phobias in addition to some of the agitated behaviors described. The Revised Memory and Behavioral Problems Checklist (RMBPC; Teri et al. 1992) assesses memory-related problems, depression problems, and disruption problems. The Neuropsychiatric Inventory (NPI; Cummings et al. 1994) assesses delusions and hallucinations, agitation and aggression, dysphoria, anxiety, apathy, disinhibition, irritability and lability, and aberrant motor activity.

There are several reasons for differentiating between agitated behaviors and related constructs. First, the different constructs assessed in the instruments mentioned may have different relationships to agitated behaviors. For example, delusions and hallucinations may cause some agitated behaviors by introducing an unrealistic reality; in contrast, depressed affect may result from the same cause as the agitated behavior, such as when undetected pain may cause both repetitive vocalizations and depression. A different relationship is sometimes present between sleep and agitation in which lack of sleep and ensuing fatigue prompt a person to move restlessly, which in turn exacerbates the need for sleep; this process may continue for a while in a vicious circle. A second reason for differentiating between agitated behaviors and related constructs stems from the fact that many of the related constructs describe internal emotional states, such as depression or anxiety, and their assessment for persons with advanced dementia may pose additional difficulties.

Another related construct frequently used to describe agitation is that of delirium. *Delirium*, according to DSM-IV-TR (American Psychiatric Association 2000), is a "disturbance of consciousness . . . manifested by a reduced clarity of awareness of the environment" in which the "ability to focus, sustain, or shift attention is impaired" (p. 136). This definition includes a change in cognition or the development of a perceptual disturbance. Delirium develops over a period of hours to days and tends to fluctuate during the course of a given day. Finally, there is evidence that delirium is caused by the direct physiological consequences of a general medical condition or a drug. Delirium is ruled out if the disturbance in consciousness, the change in cognition, or the perceptual disturbance is accounted for by dementia. Delirium can, however, be superimposed on dementia when additional symptoms of short duration are noted that are above and beyond those accounted for by the dementia and are associated with a medical condition.

Delirium is frequently accompanied by restlessness and other problem behaviors. In this way, some agitated behaviors may be accounted for by delirium. An example of such an occurrence was demonstrated in an observational study of agitation in which the prevalence of agitated behaviors increased during the time three nursing home residents had an infection (i.e., before antibiotic treatment) (Cohen-Mansfield et al. 1994). However, for a true assessment of delirium, a decline in the patients' consciousness level and cognitive level would need to be documented. In this case, their initial cognitive level was extremely compromised (their scores on the Brief Cognitive Ratings Scale were 6.6, 6.4, and 6.9, where 1 indicates normal functioning and 7 indicates a complete decline). Cohen-Mansfield et al. (1990b) also suggested that pain and chronic disease play a role in at least some types of agitated behaviors in which there is no documented rapid development of symptoms or change in cognition. Therefore, the concept of delirium is found to be of limited use in settings where most disease is chronic rather than acute. Instead, it is preferable to look for possible medical causes of agitated behaviors. Furthermore, a sudden increase in problem behavior, whether accompanied by cognitive change or not, needs to be examined as an indicator of possible medical change and pain (Marzinski 1991).

Subtypes of Problem Behaviors

Even when the domain of problem behaviors is agreed on, some controversy remains as to whether it is one construct or is composed of several subtypes. Based on factor analyses in both a senior day care population and a nursing home population, Cohen-Mansfield et al. (1995a) described problem behaviors as four subtypes: physically aggressive, physically nonaggressive, verbally aggressive, and verbally nonaggressive. These subtypes can be described as occurring on two dimensions: aggressive–nonaggressive and physical–verbal, as delineated in Figure 1–1.

Whereas the behaviors within each subtype tend to co-occur (e.g., the person who paces tends also to handle things inappropriately, such as by moving things from place to place), the subtypes are not independent (Cohen-Mansfield and Werner 1998). Because of the interrelationship among the subtypes, the original factor analysis by Cohen-Mansfield et al. (1989) identified three types of agitation—physically nonaggressive agitation, physically aggressive agitation, and verbal/vocal agitation—rather than four types. For this reason, research frequently has been conducted with three rather than four types, and thus correlates are frequently described in terms of three types.

Rating Scale for Agitated Behaviors

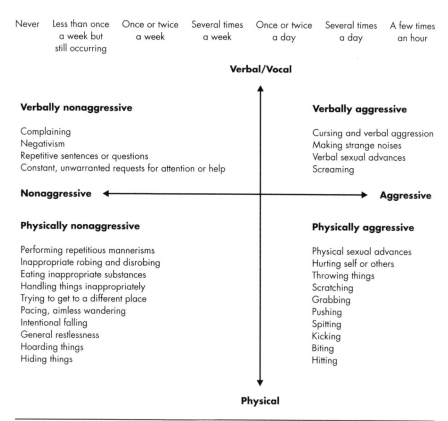

Never   Less than once   Once or twice   Several times   Once or twice   Several times   A few times
         a week but   a week   a week   a day   a day   an hour
         still occurring

Verbal/Vocal

Verbally nonaggressive

Complaining
Negativism
Repetitive sentences or questions
Constant, unwarranted requests for attention or help

Verbally aggressive

Cursing and verbal aggression
Making strange noises
Verbal sexual advances
Screaming

Nonaggressive ← → **Aggressive**

Physically nonaggressive

Performing repetitious mannerisms
Inappropriate robing and disrobing
Eating inappropriate substances
Handling things inappropriately
Trying to get to a different place
Pacing, aimless wandering
Intentional falling
General restlessness
Hoarding things
Hiding things

Physically aggressive

Physical sexual advances
Hurting self or others
Throwing things
Scratching
Grabbing
Pushing
Spitting
Kicking
Biting
Hitting

Physical

Figure 1–1   Agitated behaviors, by subgroup, along two dimensions: Cohen-Mansfield Agitation Inventory.

Source.   Reprinted from Cohen-Mansfield J: "Approaches to the Management of Disruptive Behavior," in *Alzheimer's Disease and Related Dementias: Strategies in Care and Research.* Edited by Rubinstein R, Lawton MP. New York, Springer, 1999. Springer Publishing Company, Inc., New York 10012. Used with permission. Copyright © Jiska Cohen-Mansfield, Ph.D., 1998. All rights reserved.

There are several reasons to accept the subtypes described here as a framework for studying agitation. First, this categorization system is based on the two factor analyses mentioned above, which were conducted in two independent populations: 408 nursing home residents and 200 participants of senior day care centers. Different research assistants administered somewhat different instruments to different caregivers, yet the results generally converged to these subtypes. Second, similar subtypes were found in other populations, including Dutch (De Jonghe and Kat 1996) and Japanese (Schreiner et al. 1999). Third, the different subtypes showed different patterns of relation with cognitive functioning (Cohen-Mansfield et al. 1995b) and different longitudinal patterns (Cohen-Mansfield and Werner 1998). Similarly, the medical and psychosocial correlates differ for the individual subtypes (Cohen-Mansfield et al. 1992a). Finally, much of the literature that has not considered subtypes has focused specifically on either aggressive behaviors, wandering behavior (sometimes including related physical nonaggressive behaviors), or verbally disruptive or noisy behaviors. These correspond well with the four-subtype typology represented in Figure 1–1.

The four-subtype typology is, however, not universally accepted, and other typologies have been suggested. One such typology is based on a factor analysis performed by Devanand et al. (1992) with 106 patients with probable Alzheimer's disease. The factors identified were disinhibition, apathy-indifference, catastrophic reactions, sundowning, and denial. At least one reason for these disparate findings is the use of different assessment instruments that encompass different domains.

Generally, the current literature is divided on the issue of whether to examine subtypes of problem behaviors. Whereas some researchers use total scores of assessment instruments, others use subtype scores. Furthermore, when examining aggressive behaviors, vocal/verbal behaviors, and physically nonaggressive behaviors, some researchers have proposed further typologies to describe these subtypes. For example, classification systems for subtypes of aggressive behaviors generally focus on the following dimensions: 1) the nature of the behavior, such as physical aggression, verbal aggression, or sexual aggression (Ryden 1988); 2) the target of the behavior (i.e., disturbing or endangering the self versus others) (Zimmer et al. 1984); 3) the degree of disruption (i.e., disturbing versus endangering) (Winger et al. 1987; Zimmer et al. 1984); or 4) the environmental conditions under which the behavior occurs (e.g., nighttime or during intimate care) (Patel and Hope 1992).

Similarly, several methods for classifying wandering behaviors have been suggested (Table 1–1). The methods demonstrate different emphases in describing the behavior, such as the reason for the behavior (e.g., caused by medication, intent to escape, need for stimulation) (Hussian 1987); the description of the actual travel route taken (e.g., direct travel, random travel, pacing, lapping) (Martino-Saltzman et al. 1991); the impact on others (e.g., trespassing) (Milke 1988); and the level of supervision and intent (i.e., purposeful or goal-directed versus aimless) (Snyder et al. 1978).

For verbally disruptive behaviors, two classification systems have been introduced. Ryan et al. (1988) developed a system with six classes of

Table 1–1. Classification systems to describe pacing and wandering behaviors

Source	Subtypes	Description
Butler and Barnett (1991)	Purposeful wanderer	Walking with apparent intent; caregiver knows person's whereabouts
	Escapist	Purposeful intent on going elsewhere, frequently from institution to home
	Aimless wanderer	Confused, purposeless walk
	Critical wanderer	Confused wanderer who leaves the premises without caregiver's knowledge
Hussian and Brown (1987)	Akathisias	Antipsychotic induced
	Exit seekers	Attempting to leave the unit or facility
	Self-stimulators	Turning doorknobs and pacing continuously
	Modelers	"Shadowing" or following other pacers
Martino-Saltzman et al. (1991)	Direct travel	Move from one location to another without diversion
	Random travel	Move in a roundabout, haphazard manner to many areas
	Pacing	Repetitive walking back and forth in a limited area
	Lapping	Repetitive walking, circling large areas
Milke (1988)	Absconding	Leaving an activity, unit, or facility
	Locomotive restlessness	Walking with no obvious purpose or destination
	Group walking	Aimless locomotion as part of a group
	Motoric restlessness	Fiddling with objects; small, repetitive muscle movements
	Navigational difficulty	Errors in finding his or her way, visual scanning of the environment
	Searching	Actively looking for objects or persons
	Trespassing	Uninvited entry into another's room
Snyder et al. (1978)	Goal directed or searching	Searching for something that is often unobtainable
	Goal directed or industrious	Drive to do things or to remain busy
	Non–goal directed	Aimlessly wandering, drawn from one stimulus to another

Source. Reprinted from Cohen-Mansfield et al.: "Wandering and Aggression," in *The Practical Handbook of Clinical Gerontology.* Edited by Carstensen LL et al. Thousand Oaks, CA, Sage, 1996, pp. 374–397. Copyright 1996, Sage Publications, Inc. Reprinted by permission of Sage Publications, Inc.

verbally disruptive behaviors: 1) noise making that appears purposeless and perseverative; 2) noise making that is a response to the environment; 3) noise making that elicits a response from the environment; 4) "chatterbox" noise making; 5) noise making caused by deafness; and 6) other noise making. Cohen-Mansfield and Werner (1997b) developed the Typology of Vocalizations (TOV), which rates problem vocalizations on four dimensions: 1) type of sound, 2) meaning/reason/content of sound, 3) timing, and 4) level of disruptiveness.

Etiology of Problem Behaviors

The importance of determining the etiology of problem behaviors lies not only in a deeper understanding of these behaviors but also in the immediate implications for treatment or prevention of the behaviors. Those who believe the behaviors result directly from brain dysfunction through disinhibition or direct neurological activation of certain behaviors (e.g., screaming) are more likely to seek pharmacological solutions. Those who attribute the behaviors to learning through differential reinforcement (e.g., behavior as a request for attention may be reinforced because attention is only given when the patient manifests the behavior) are likely to use a change in contingencies (e.g., reinforcing appropriate behavior and ignoring inappropriate behavior) and other behavioral interventions. Others have suggested that problem behaviors in people with dementia may result from overstimulation that the patient cannot process because of his or her cognitive incapacity. Researchers who embrace this approach study the effect of an environment with reduced stimulation. The opposing view—that problem behaviors result from understimulation and sensory deprivation—has also been proposed, and the treatment approach for this etiology involves either increasing the level of stimulation for the patient and ensuring that the type of stimulation can be processed (i.e., that it is matched to the individual's abilities and deficits) or accommodating the self-stimulatory behavior emitted by the patient.

Generally, there is consensus that behavioral problems are related to cognitive impairment, but lower levels of some behaviors are also manifested in people who do not have dementia (Koss et al. 1997). The relationship between problem behaviors and stage of dementia varies across each syndrome (Cohen-Mansfield and Deutsch 1996; Cohen-Mansfield et al. 1990a; Micas et al. 1995). Physically aggressive behavior is more likely to be manifested by individuals with severe cognitive impairment. Physically nonaggressive behavior tends to increase in prevalence with the deterioration of cognitive functioning. Verbally nonaggressive behavior increases in the early stages of dementia and then either increases to middle levels or plateaus and decreases in the end stages of dementia. Verbally aggressive behavior, like physically aggressive behavior, tends to increase only in the late stages of dementia, although generally earlier than physically aggressive behavior (Cohen-Mansfield et al. 1995b).

Models for the Causes of Problem Behaviors

The consistent relationship between cognitive impairment and problem behaviors naturally raises the question of what role dementia plays in causing these behaviors (e.g., Marx et al. 1990; Meddaugh 1987; Naesman et al. 1993; Patel and Hope 1992; Ryden 1988; Swearer et al. 1988; and Winger et al. 1987). Theories relating to this issue can be divided into four general categories, the first of which pertains to the direct impact of dementia; the other three focus on factors that interact with dementia or with the context of dementia. These are summarized below.

Model I: Direct impact of dementia. The direct-impact model (see Figure 1–2) is based on two premises: 1) problem behaviors result directly from pathophysiological changes in the brain, and 2) severe organic brain deterioration results in behavioral disinhibition.

Model II: Unmet needs. According to the unmet needs model, the dementia process results in a decreased ability to meet one's needs because of a decreased ability to communicate those needs and to provide for oneself (see Figure 1–3). Needs may pertain to pain, health, or physical discomfort; mental discomfort evident in affective states such as depression, anxiety, and frustration; lack of social contacts; uncomfortable environmental conditions; or inadequate level of stimulation (i.e., too low, too high, inappropriate).

Model III: Behavioral. According to the behavioral model (see Figure 1–4), the problem behavior is controlled by its antecedents and consequences. Many problem behaviors are learned through reinforcement by staff members who provide attention when a problem behavior is displayed (ABC model: Antecedents lead to Behavior that leads to Consequences, i.e., antecedents operate through stimulus control, and the consequences reinforce behavior or reinforce certain behaviors related to specific antecedent stimuli).

Model IV: Environmental vulnerability. According to this model, the dementia process results in greater vulnerability to the environment and a lower threshold at which stimuli affect behavior. Thus, a stimulus that may be appropriate for a cognitively intact person may result in overreaction in a cognitively impaired person.

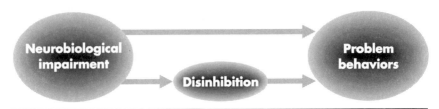

Figure 1–2   Direct impact of dementia model.

Source.   Copyright © Jiska Cohen-Mansfield, Ph.D., 1998. All rights reserved.

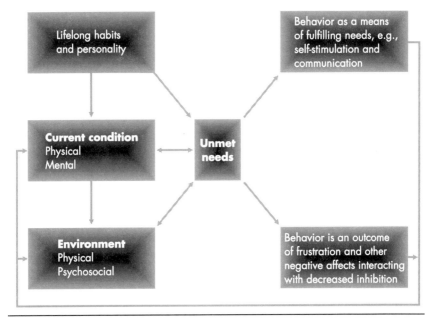

Figure 1–3   Unmet needs model.

Source.   Reprinted from Cohen-Mansfield J, Taylor L: "Assessing and Understanding Agitated Behaviors in Older Adults," in *Behaviors in Dementia: Best Practices for Successful Management.* Edited by Kaplan M, Hoffman SB. Baltimore, MD, Health Professions Press, 1998. Copyright © Jiska Cohen-Mansfield, Ph.D., 1998. All rights reserved.

These models are not mutually exclusive and can be interactive. For example, an environmental vulnerability (Model IV) may make a person with dementia more susceptible to environmental antecedents and consequences (Model III). Environmental vulnerability may produce an unmet need (Model II) when normal levels of stimulation are perceived as over-stimulation, or a behavior may be the result of both frustration resulting

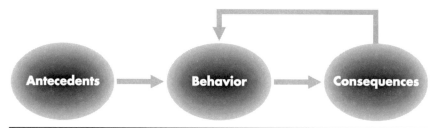

Figure 1–4 Behavioral model.
Source. Copyright © Jiska Cohen-Mansfield, Ph.D., 1998. All rights reserved.

from unmet needs (Model II) and disinhibition in manifesting this frustration (Model I). Furthermore, different models may account for different behaviors in different people. The evidence for each of these models is summarized below.

Direct Impact of Dementia: Does Dementia Directly Affect Problem Behaviors Through Neurological Mechanisms?

A relationship between abnormalities in neurotransmission and behavior problems has been suggested by Palmer et al. (1988), who discovered decreased postmortem cortical serotonin levels among agitated individuals. Similarly, Schneider et al. (1988) found reduced platelet tritiated imipramine binding, a marker of serotonin dysfunction, among agitated patients with dementia. In contrast, Lawlor et al. (1989) conducted a study that involved the administration of a serotonin agonist and found agitation to increase. Other neurotransmitters have been examined as well. For example, Brane et al. (1989) reported increased cerebrospinal fluid levels of 4-methoxy-5-hydroxyphenylglycol, the major metabolite of norepinephrine among agitated individuals, and Russo-Neustadt and Cotman (1997) found that agitated elderly patients had more adrenergic receptors in the cerebellum. Furthermore, a nonsignificant trend was reported by Sweet et al. (1997) for a relationship between treatment with plasma homovanillic acid, a dopamine metabolite, and increased agitation. Positron emission tomography (PET) studies have also found behavior problems to be related to selective impairment of glucose utilization in the frontal region (Chase et al. 1987; Kumar et al. 1990) and to hypometabolism and selective reduction in glucose utilization in the frontal and temporal regions (Sultzer et al. 1995). Cacabelos et al. (1996; 1997) did not find statistically significant differences in behavioral problems among different apolipoprotein genotypes. These studies varied in the methodologies used, types of behavioral problems included, samples, and results. Further research is

needed to elucidate the relationship between behavior and pathophysiological mechanisms.

Unmet Needs Interact With Dementia

According to the unmet needs model, problem behaviors result from an
imbalance in the interaction between lifelong habits and personality, current physical and mental states, and less-than-optimal environmental conditions (Figure 1–3). Most unmet needs arise because of dementia-related
impairments in both communication and the ability to use the environment appropriately to accommodate needs. Agitated behaviors result
from unmet needs in one of two ways: 1) the behavior represents a desire
to alleviate the need either by meeting it (e.g., pacing to alleviate boredom
and understimulation) or by communicating it (e.g., making repetitive vocalizations), or 2) the behavior may signal the outcome of having an unmet
need by communicating distress, frustration, or pain. Examples of specific
unmet needs leading to agitation are described below.

- **Pain, ill health, and/or physical discomfort.** Physical pain and ill health
  factors have been associated with verbal and vocal forms of behavior
  problems (Cohen-Mansfield et al. 1990b). Hurley et al. (1992) reported
  an increase in negative vocalizations among patients experiencing fe-
  vers. Similarly, pain medications relieved behavior problems in a study
  by Douzjian et al. (1998). The behavior problem may be a direct manifestation of the discomfort—a natural response to pain—and may be exacerbated in patients who have an impaired ability to communicate.
  Alternatively, the vocally disruptive behavior may be an attempt by a
  cognitively impaired individual to communicate the discomfort.
    The relationship between health and physically aggressive behavior
  is less clear, but a positive association between aggressive behavior and
  urinary tract infections has been reported (Ryden and Bossenmaier
  1988). In contrast, people who engage in physically nonaggressive behavior (e.g., pacing) have been reported to have fewer medical diagnoses than other nursing home residents and to have better appetites
  (Cohen-Mansfield et al. 1990b). However, some people who pace suffer
  from akathesia, an inner sense of restlessness that is caused by a neurodegenerative disease or by an extrapyramidal reaction to an antipsychotic or other drug (Mutch 1992).
    Sleep disturbance and fatigue are other aspects of health that have
  been linked to problem behaviors (Cohen-Mansfield and Marx 1990;
  Cohen-Mansfield et al. 1995c). The impairment of circadian rhythms
  that is characteristic of Alzheimer's disease (Bliwise 1993) may also be

related to behavior problems. In particular, an increase in behavior problems, such as in elderly individuals with dementia, that occurs in the evening hours, beginning at a time near sunset, has been termed *sundowning* (Bliwise 1994).

- **Mental discomfort evident in affective states such as depression, anxiety, and frustration.** These affective processes may themselves be the result of neurobiological changes, lifelong problems, the individual's confrontation with his or her decreasing abilities, or various unmet needs. Research revealed a relationship between verbal/vocal problem behaviors and depressed affect, but similar results were not uncovered with physically nonaggressive behaviors (Cohen-Mansfield and Marx 1988). This finding may be related to the higher prevalence of physical pain and the relatively higher level of cognitive functioning among those who manifest verbal/vocal agitation. Therefore, they are better able to communicate their moods (via complaints or other negative comments) to caregivers than persons manifesting other types of behavior problems. Several reports have linked aggressive behaviors with depressed affect (e.g., McShane et al. 2000; Menon et al. 2001).

- **Need for social contacts.** Cohen-Mansfield and Werner (1995) found that verbal/vocal problem behaviors, as well as some physically nonaggressive behaviors other than pacing and wandering, tended to increase in frequency when nursing home residents manifesting these problem behaviors were alone and to decrease when residents were with other people. Similarly, such behaviors decreased when staffing levels increased. These findings suggest that loneliness or the need for social contact may be at the root of problem behaviors. Supporting this idea is an intervention study (Cohen-Mansfield and Werner 1997a) in which social interaction was more beneficial in decreasing verbal and vocal problem behaviors than the mere provision of pleasant stimuli, such as music.

- **Uncomfortable environmental conditions.** In an observational study of the nursing home environment, most problem behaviors tended to increase when it was cold at night, and requests for attention increased when it was hot during the day (Cohen-Mansfield and Werner 1995). These findings suggest that discomfort may cause some behavior problems.

- **Inadequate level of stimulation (i.e., too low, too high, or inappropriate) and/or sensory deprivation.** Problem behaviors have been attributed to overstimulation that cannot be processed because of the dementia (Cleary et al. 1988; Johnson 1989; Meyer et al. 1992). An observational study of a nursing home conducted by Cohen-Mansfield et al.

(1992b) did not support this hypothesis; rather, their observations revealed the nursing home to be a relatively monotonous place where routine is the rule and activities and stimulation are infrequent (Cohen-Mansfield et al. 1992a). Most problem behaviors increased when the older person was inactive and decreased when structured activities were offered (Cohen-Mansfield and Werner 1995). Our position is therefore in opposition to the overstimulation hypothesis. We contend that problem behaviors result from understimulation and sensory deprivation—the person with dementia has reduced ability to obtain stimulation and process it. He or she also may have vision and hearing deficits that further reduce the ability to process stimuli. Many nursing homes in which persons with dementia reside offer few activities or other positive stimuli. All of these factors result in a state of sensory deprivation to which the person responds with either self-stimulation or with behaviors that manifest discontent because of this unmet need for stimulation. Studies on social deprivation in younger populations have shown that sensory deprivation can result in hallucinations and perceptual distortions, which may in turn cause problem behaviors. Even without hallucinations or perceptual changes, sensory deprivation may evoke emotions of fear, loneliness, and boredom, all resulting in the manifestation of problem behaviors. Several studies have shown that providing sensory stimulation to nursing home residents decreases behavioral disturbances in general and vocally disruptive behaviors in particular (Birchmore and Clague 1983; Mayers and Griffin 1990; Zachow 1984).

Delusions and hallucinations, regardless of their cause, provide inappropriate internal stimuli that may result in problem behaviors. The relationship between problem behaviors and delusions or hallucinations has been documented repeatedly (Cohen-Mansfield et al. 1998; Deutsch et al. 1991; Lachs et al. 1992; Steiger et al. 1991).

Behavioral Model

According to the behavioral model, problem behavior is controlled by its antecedents and consequences. Problem behaviors are operants, learned through reinforcement; attention to the patient is given by caregivers when the problem behavior is displayed. Within the social vacuum of the nursing home, any attention is a potent reinforcer. Other types of learning processes, such as those involved in stimulus control, may also be operating. In a description of a 70-year-old blind woman, Birchmore and Clague (1983) observed that the patient screamed more when the nurses spoke to her. Findings collected by Cohen-Mansfield et al. (1992c) in the nursing home did not support this model. Most behaviors were not triggered by any observable incident, and most did not receive any reaction. The highest rates of triggering events and reactions were for aggressive behaviors, which seemed to be triggered in 26% of the cases and responded to in 43%. Rates were less than half that for other behaviors. Of course, it is still possible that behaviors are reinforced and maintained on a low reinforcement schedule, but this schedule would be very low for most behaviors. Furthermore, this model relies on the assumption that learning can occur in dementia, when the mechanisms responsible for learning are those specifically impaired in dementia. Some case reports and small studies have reported successful use of behavioral treatments; however, given that the behavioral treatment usually involved giving the elderly patient increased attention, the provision of attention (thereby fulfilling social needs) rather than the contingency of attention as a consequence of the behavior may be the factor responsible for the change in behavior. The poor control used in most studies does not allow for proper distinction between these possibilities. Furthermore, there are reports, albeit unpublished, of behavioral treatment failure or even exacerbation of behavioral problems with treatment (Lewin 1996).

Environmental Vulnerability Model

The concept of person–environment congruence (French et al. 1974; Kahana 1982) and the press–competence model (Lawton and Nahemow 1973) suggest that for optimal functioning, a match is needed between the person's needs and abilities and the demands of the environment as related to those needs and abilities. For any level of competence, there is a range of environmental demands that is favorable. Furthermore, the environmental docility hypothesis (Lawton and Simon 1968) states that as personal competence decreases, the environment becomes a more potent determinant of behavioral outcome. Fitting these theoretical perspectives are both the overstimulation and the understimulation hypotheses described earlier. Research results support the understimulation concept—that is, the idea that a lack of sufficient and appropriate stimulation is the cause of certain types of problem behaviors and that the environment must be modified to match an individual's stimulation needs and capabilities.

Etiology of Problem Behaviors by Subtypes of Problems

Different types of problem behaviors are related to different needs. Correlational studies forming the basis for inference of needs are summarized in Table 1–2. Verbal behaviors are related to discomfort, loneliness, and suf-

Table 1-2. Personal and environmental correlates of the different types of agitation

Correlates	Vocal/verbal behaviors	Physically nonaggressive behaviors	Aggressive behaviors
Personal attributes			
Gender	Female		Male
Cognitive	Cognitive impairment	Moderate to severe impairment	Severe cognitive impairment
Health	Poor health or pain	Relatively good health	
Affect	Depressed affect		
Sleep	Sleep problems	Sleep problems	Sleep problems
Stress		Past stress	
Social function	Poor quality of social relations		Poor quality of social relations
Environmental			
Social	Alone	Some others around	Directed more at staff
Location	In own room	In public spaces or corridors	In own room
Activities	No activities	No activities	
Time	Evening or night	All day	Evening, lunch
Environmental		Normal environmental conditions (e.g., temperature, noise)	Cold or noisy at night
Possible needs	Loneliness	Self-stimulation	Evasion of discomfort
	Fears		Attempt to communicate need
	Pain		
	Depression		

fering. Physically nonaggressive behaviors are not related to suffering, occur under normal conditions, and appear to be adaptive in providing stimulation. Aggressive behaviors are those least explained by the unmet needs model, but some behaviors appear to be the result of discomfort or an effort to communicate.

Conclusions

Problem behaviors are a complex phenomenon affected by an interaction of cognitive impairment, physical health, mental health, past habits and personality, and environmental factors. As such, agitated behaviors vary among individuals. Several subtypes of problem behaviors are differentially related to those factors. These subtypes are useful in guiding the formulation of an individualized treatment plan. Such a plan would involve several stages: 1) hypothesize which need underlies the agitated behaviors; 2) characterize the way in which the behavior results from the need (Does the behavior attempt to accommodate the need? Does it express discomfort? Does it attempt to communicate the need?); and 3) provide an intervention that provides for the unmet need or, if the behavior itself alleviates the need, provide a method by which the behavior can be accommodated. The goals of this plan are to improve the quality of life for the patient and to reduce the burden on caregivers.

References

American Psychiatric Association: Diagnostic and Statistical Manual of Mental Disorders, 4th Edition Text Revision. Washington, DC, American Psychiatric Association, 2000

Bliwise DL: Sleep in normal aging and dementia. Sleep 16:40–81, 1993

Bliwise DL: What is sundowning? J Am Geriatr Soc 42:1009–1011, 1994

Birchmore T, Clague S: A behavioural approach to reduce shouting. Nursing Times 79:37–39, 1983

Brane G, Gottfries CG, Blennow K, et al: Monoamine metabolism in cerebrospinal fluid and behavioral ratings in patients with early and late onset Alzheimer's disease. Alzheimer Dis Assoc Disord 3:148–156, 1989

Butler JP, Barnett CA: Window of wandering. Geriatr Nurs 12:226–227, 1991

Cacabelos R, Rodriguez B, Carrera C, et al: APOE-related frequency of cognitive and noncognitive symptoms in dementia. Method Find Exp Clin Pharmacol 18:693–706, 1996

Cacabelos R, Rodriguez B, Carrera C., et al: Behavioral changes associated with different apolipoprotein E genotypes in dementia. Alzheimer Dis Assoc Disord 11(suppl):27–34, 1997

Chase TN, Burrows GH, Mohr E: Cortical glucose utilization patterns in primary degenerative dementias of the anterior and posterior type. Arch Gerontol Geriatr 6:289–297, 1987

Cleary TA, Clamon C, Price M, et al: A reduced simulation unit: effects on patients with Alzheimer's disease and related disorders. Gerontologist 28:511–514, 1988

Cohen-Mansfield J, Billig N: Agitated behaviors in the elderly: a conceptual review. J Am Geriatr Soc 34:711–721, 1986

Cohen-Mansfield J, Deutsch L: Agitation: subtypes and their mechanisms. Semin Clin Neuropsychiatry 1:325–339, 1996

Cohen-Mansfield J, Marx MS: Relationship between depression and agitation in nursing home residents. Comprehensive Gerontology B 2:141–146, 1988

Cohen-Mansfield J, Marx MS: The relationship between sleep disturbances and agitation in a nursing home. Journal of Aging and Health 2:153–165, 1990

Cohen-Mansfield J, Werner P: Environmental influences on agitation: an integrative summary of an observational study. American Journal of Alzheimer's Care and Related Disorders and Research 10:32–39, 1995

Cohen-Mansfield J, Werner P: Management of verbally disruptive behaviors in the nursing home. J Gerontol Med Sci 52(suppl A):M369–M377, 1997a

Cohen-Mansfield J, Werner P: Typology of verbally disruptive behaviors in the nursing home. Int J Geriatr Psychiatry 12:1079–1091, 1997b

Cohen-Mansfield J, Werner P: Longitudinal changes in behavioral problems in old age: a study in an adult day care population. J Gerontol Med Sci 53A:M65–M71, 1998

Cohen-Mansfield J, Marx MS, Rosenthal AS: A description of agitation in a nursing home. J Gerontol Med Sci 44:M77–M84, 1989

Cohen-Mansfield J, Marx M, Rosenthal AS: Dementia and agitation in nursing home residents: how are they related? Psychology and Aging 5:3–8, 1990a

Cohen-Mansfield J, Billig N, Lipson S, et al: Medical correlates of agitation in nursing home residents. Gerontology 36:150–158, 1990b

Cohen-Mansfield J, Marx MS, Werner P: Agitation in elderly persons: an integrative report of findings in a nursing home. International Psychogeriatrics 4(suppl):221–240, 1992a

Cohen-Mansfield J, Marx MS, Werner P: Observational data on time use and behavior problems in the nursing home. Journal of Applied Gerontology 11:111–121, 1992b

Cohen-Mansfield J, Werner P, Marx MS: The social environment of the agitated nursing home resident. Int J Geriatr Psychiatry 7:789–798, 1992c

Cohen-Mansfield J, Werner P, Marx MS: The impact of infection on agitation: three case studies in the nursing home. American Journal of Alzheimer's Care and Related Disorders and Research July/August:30–34, 1994

Cohen-Mansfield J, Werner P, Watson V, et al: Agitation in participants of adult day care centers: the experiences of relatives and staff members. International Psychogeriatrics 7:447–458, 1995a

Cohen-Mansfield J, Culpepper WJ, Werner P: The relationship between cognitive function and agitation in senior day care participants. Int J Geriatr 10:585–595, 1995b

Cohen-Mansfield J, Werner P, Freedman L: Sleep and agitation in agitated nursing home residents: an observational study. Sleep 18:674–680, 1995c

Cohen-Mansfield J, Taylor L, Werner P: Delusions and hallucinations in an adult day care population: a longitudinal study. Am J Geriatr Psychiatry 6:104–121, 1998

Cummings JL, Mega M, Gray K, et al: The neuropsychiatric inventory: comprehensive assessment of psychopathology in dementia. Neurology 44:2308–2314, 1994

De Jonghe JFM, Kat MG: Factor structure and validity of the Dutch version of the Cohen-Mansfield Agitation Inventory (CMAI-D). J Am Geriatr Soc 44:888–889, 1996

Deutsch LH, Bylsma FW, Rovner BW, et al: Psychosis and physical aggression in probable Alzheimer's disease. Am J Psychiatry 148:1159–1163, 1991

Devanand DP, Brockington CD, Moody BJ, et al: Behavioral syndromes in Alzheimer's disease. International Psychogeriatrics 4(suppl):161–185, 1992

Douzjian M, Wilson C, Shultz M, et al: A program to use pain control medication to reduce psychotropic drug use in residents with difficult behavior. Ann Long-Term Care 6:174–179, 1998

French JPR, Rodgers W, Cobbs S: Adjustment as person–environment fit, in Coping and Adaptation. Edited by Coelho GV, Hamburg DA, Adams JE. New York, Basic Books, 1974, pp 316–333

Hurley A, Volicer B, Hanrahan P, et al: Assessment of discomfort in advanced Alzheimer patients. Res Nurs Health 15:369–377, 1992

Hussian RA, Brown DC: Use of two-dimensional grid patterns to limit hazardous ambulation in demented patients. J Gerontol 42:558–560, 1987

Johnson CJ: Sociological intervention through developing low stimulus Alzheimer's wings in nursing homes. American Journal of Alzheimer's Care and Related Disorder and Research 4:33–41, 1989

Kahana E: A congruence model of person-environment interaction, in Aging and the Environment: Theoretical Approaches. Edited by Lawton MP, Windley PG, Byerts TO. New York, Springer, 1982, pp 97–121

Koss E, Weiner M, Ernesto C, et al: Assessing patterns of agitation in Alzheimer's disease patients with the Cohen-Mansfield Agitation Inventory: The Alzheimer's Disease Cooperative Study. Alzheimer Dis Assoc Disord 11(suppl):45–50, 1997

Kumar A, Schapiro MB, Haxby JV, et al: Cerebral metabolic and cognitive studies in dementia with frontal lobe behavioral features. J Psychiatr Res 24:97–109, 1990

Lachs MS, Becker M, Siegal, AP, et al: Delusions and behavioral disturbances in cognitively impaired elderly persons. J Am Gerontol Soc 40:768–773, 1992

Lawlor BA, Sunderland T, Mellow AM, et al: Hyperresponsivity to the serotonin agonist m-chlorophenylpiperazine in Alzheimer's disease. Arch Gen Psychiatry 46:542–549, 1989

Lawton MP, Nahemow L: Ecology and the aging process, in Psychology of Adult Development and Aging. Edited by Eisdorfer C, Lawton MP. Washington, DC, American Psychological Association, 1973, pp 619–674

Lawton MP, Simon B: The ecology of social relationships in housing for the elderly. Gerontologist 8:108–115, 1968

Lewin L: Disruptive vocalizations in nursing home residents: treatment, successes, and failure. Presentation to the American Psychological Association 104th convention, Toronto, Canada, August 1996

Marx MS, Cohen-Mansfield J, Werner P: A profile of the aggressive nursing home resident. Behavior, Health, and Aging 1:65–73, 1990

Martino-Saltzman D, Blasch BB, Morris RD, et al: Travel behavior of nursing home residents perceived as wanderers and nonwanderers. Gerontologist 31:666–672, 1991

Marzinski L: The tragedy of dementia: clinically assessing pain in the confused, nonverbal elderly. J Gerontol Nurs 17:25–28, 1991

Mayers K, Griffin M: The play project: use of stimulus objects with demented patients. J Gerontol Nurs 16:32–37, 1990

McShane R, Cohen-Mansfield, Werner P: Predictors of aggressive behaviors. Res Pract Alz Dis 3:183–188, 2000

Meddaugh DI: Aggressive and nonaggressive nursing home patients. Gerontologist 27:127A, 1987

Menon AS, Gruber-Baldini AL, Hebel JR, et al: Relationships between aggressive behaviors and depression among nursing home residents with dementia. Int J Geriatr Psychiatry 16:139–146, 2001

Meyer DL, Dorbacker B, O'Rourke J, et al: Effects of a "quiet week" intervention on behavior in an Alzheimer boarding home. American Journal of Alzheimer's Care and Related Disorders and Research July/August 7:2–7, 1992

Micas M, Ousset PJ, Vellas B: Evaluation des troubles dur comportement. Presentation de L'echelle de Cohen-Mansfield. La Revue Française de Psychiatrie et de Psychologie Medicale 7:151–154, 1995

Milke DL: Wandering in dementia: behavioral observations. Gerontologist 28(special issue):47, 1988

Mutch WJ: Parkinsonism and other movement disorders, in Textbook of Geriatric Medicine and Gerontology. Edited by Brocklehurst JC, Tallis RC, Fillit HM. New York, Churchill Livingstone, 1992, pp 565–593

Naesman B, Bucht G, Eriksson S, et al: Behavioral symptoms in the institutionalized elderly: relationship to dementia. Int J Geriatr Psychiatry 8:843–849, 1993

Palmer AM, Stratman GC, Procter AW, et al: Possible neurotransmitter basis of behavioral changes in Alzheimer's disease. Ann Neurol 34:616–620, 1988

Patel V, Hope RA: A rating scale for aggressive behaviour in the elderly: the RAGE. Psychol Med 22:211–221, 1992

Reisberg B, Borenstein J, Franssen E, et al: BEHAVE-AD: a clinical rating scale for the assessment of pharmacologically remediable symptomology in Alzheimer's disease, in Alzheimer's Disease: Problems and Perspectives. Edited by Altman HJ. New York, Plenum Press, 1987, pp 1–16

Russo-Neustadt A, Cotman CW: Adrenergic receptors in Alzheimer's disease brain: selective increases in the cerebella of aggressive patients. J Neurosci 17:5573–5580, 1997

Ryan DP, Tainsh SM, Kolodny V, et al: Noise-making among the elderly in long term care. Gerontologist 28:369–371, 1988

Ryden MB: Aggressive behavior in persons with dementia living in the community. Alzheimer Dis Assoc Disord 2:342–355, 1988

Ryden M, Bossenmaier M: Aggressive behaviors in cognitively impaired nursing home residents. Gerontologist 28(suppl A):179, 1988

Schneider LS, Severson JA, Chui HC, et al: Platelet tritiated imipramine binding and MAO activity in Alzheimer's patients with agitation and delusions. Psychiatry Res 25:311–322, 1988

Schreiner AS, Yamamoto E, Shiotani H: Behavioral syndromes and characteristics of dementia patients in a sample of nursing homes in western Japan. Gerontologist 39(special issue 1):332, 1999

Snyder LH, Ruppicht R, Pyrek J, et al: Wandering. Gerontologist 18:272–280, 1978

Steiger MJ, Quinn NP, Toone B, et al: Off-period screaming accompanying motor fluctuations in Parkinson's disease. Movement Disorders 6:89–90, 1991

Sultzer DL, Mahler ME, Mandelkern MA, et al: The relationship between psychiatric symptoms and regional cortical metabolism in Alzheimer's disease. J Neuropsychiatry Clin Neurosci 7:476–484, 1995

Swearer JM, Drachman DA, O'Donnell BF, et al: Troublesome and disruptive behaviors in dementia: relationships to diagnosis and disease severity. J Am Geriatr Soc 36:784–790, 1988

Sweet RA, Pollock BG, Mulsant BH, et al: Association of plasma homovanillic acid with behavioral symptoms in patients diagnosed with dementia: a preliminary report. Biol Psychiatry 42:1016–1023, 1997

Teri L, Traux P, Logsdon R, et al: Assessment of behavioral problems in dementia: the revised memory and behavior problems checklist. Psychol Aging 7:622–631, 1992

Winger J, Schirm V, Stewart D: Aggressive behaviors in long-term care. J Psychosoc Nurs 25:28–33, 1987

Zachow KM: Helen, can you hear me? J Gerontol Nurs 10:18–22, 1984

Zimmer JG, Watson N, Treat A: Behavioral problems among patients in skilled nursing facilities. Am J Public Health 74:1118–1121, 1984

CHAPTER 2

Epidemiology of Agitation

Karin Barkin, M.D.
Jacobo E. Mintzer, M.D.

Understanding the epidemiology of agitation is critical to providing for the current and future needs of patients with dementia and of their caregivers. In this chapter we review the epidemiology of agitation in demented populations, specifically the epidemiology of agitation in patients with dementia as a function of three different characteristics: level of cognitive impairment, demographics, and patient settings.

Level of Cognitive Impairment

Alzheimer's Disease

Although it is generally observed that most individuals with Alzheimer's disease (AD) exhibit behavioral symptoms, studies are in less accord with respect to the relationship between agitation and cognitive impairment. Burns et al. (1990) studied 178 subjects with probable or possible AD for behavioral disturbances. They found that 19.7% of the patients exhibited physically aggressive behavior, 18.5% were wandering, and 35.6% went into rages. The study identified a positive correlation between the severity of dementia and the occurrence of behavioral disturbances.

Cooper et al. (1990) examined 680 patients with probable AD and found that agitation was associated with declining Mini-Mental State Examination (MMSE) scores. The prevalence of agitated behaviors increased from 37.5% in patients with mild dementia to 66.5% in patients with severe dementia. Teri et al. (1988) also reported an increasing prevalence of behavioral disturbances associated with decreasing mental status in patients with AD. In their study, 10% of patients presenting with mild dementia (as measured by the MMSE), 27% with moderate dementia, and 38% with severe dementia were agitated; 18%, 22%, and 50%, respectively, exhibited wandering; and 60%, 40%, and 50%, respectively, exhibited restlessness. In this group of outpatients, there was an association between degree of cognitive impairment and agitation and wandering. In contrast, restlessness did not increase with greater cognitive impairment; it was common to all levels of impairment and affected approximately half of all patients.

Eisdorfer et al. (1992) found that although the patients displayed agitation at all stages, a statistically significant increase in agitation occurred in the late stages of AD. They reported agitation in 4% of patients with very mild AD, 13.8% with mild AD, 40% with mild to moderate AD, 35.1% with moderate AD, 47.8% with moderate to severe AD, and 62.5% with severe AD.

Mega et al. (1996) assessed behaviors in outpatients with probable AD and found that 47% with mild dementia (as measured by the MMSE), 55% with moderate dementia, and 85% with severe dementia had agitation; 12%, 30%, and 84%, respectively, exhibited aberrant motor behavior. In patients with mild cognitive impairment, agitation correlated with anxiety, disinhibition, and irritability. In moderately impaired patients, agitation was associated with delusions and hallucinations, and in the most severely impaired patients, no correlation with other neuropsychiatric symptoms was identified. Moreover, findings from a subsequent study of 56 patients led Teri et al. (1989) also to report an increasing prevalence of behavioral disturbances associated with decreasing mental status in patients with AD.

In contrast, Hamel et al. (1990) found that level of cognitive deterioration did not predict aggression in patients with dementia residing in the community. In their study of 75 outpatients with AD, Aarsland et al. (1996) found that aggressive and nonaggressive patients did not differ in their severity of dementia.

Although further research may provide conclusive evidence of a correlation between the degree of cognitive impairment and agitation behaviors, the divergent conclusions suggested by current data indicate the need for additional empirical study.

Other Dementias

Most cases of dementia are accounted for by AD. Multi-infarcts or other cerebrovascular disorders cause another significant subtype of dementia.

The remaining 15% of cases includes dementias associated with well-recognized neurological disorders.

Sultzer et al. (1993) compared the profile of symptoms in patients with multi-infarct dementia with that of patients with AD. They did not find any significant difference in symptoms of agitation when the two groups were matched for severity of cognitive impairment, age, and educational background. Cohen et al. (1993) compared the occurrence of psychiatric symptoms in a large group of community-residing participants who met clinical diagnostic criteria for AD or multi-infarct dementia as well as mixed dementia (AD and multi-infarct dementia). They found that 29.2% of the patients with AD, 28.9% of the patients with multi-infarct dementia, and 27.9% of the patients with mixed dementia displayed agitation. In fact, agitation and depression were the two most common psychiatric conditions in patients with AD or multi-infarct dementia. Harris et al. (1994) compared the behavioral symptoms of 61 multi-infarct dementia cases with 86 multi-infarct control subjects without dementia and found that 40.7% of patients with multi-infarct dementia and 19% of the control group had agitation. Swearer et al. (1988) studied 126 subjects from a dementia research clinic in a department of neurology. The frequency of angry outbursts was 51%, and the frequency of assaultive or violent behavior was 21%. There was no difference in frequency among the three diagnostic groups of AD, multi-infarct dementia, and mixed dementia.

Levy et al. (1996b) compared 17 patients with a clinical diagnosis of frontotemporal dementia with 30 patients with a clinical diagnosis of AD. There were no statistically significant differences between the subscale scores for agitation. Mendez et al. (1993) reviewed the clinical records of 21 patients with pathologically confirmed Pick's disease and matched them with 42 patients who had confirmed AD. He found that aggression was common in both groups.

Very few published reports explore abnormal behavior in progressive supranuclear palsy; most are single-case studies. Patients with progressive supranuclear palsy had significantly less agitation than patients with AD (Litvan et al. 1996). In addition, few studies examine the relationship between behavioral problems and dementias other than AD.

Demographic Groups

No clinical studies have definitively illuminated the specific issue of the relationship between agitation and patient demographics. Reisberg et al. (1987) did a chart review of 57 severely impaired outpatients with AD. They found that patients with behavioral symptoms did not differ significantly from those without behavioral problems in respect to age or gender. Additionally, a study conducted by Aarsland et al. (1996) assessed 75 outpatients with possible or probable AD. These investigators found that neither age nor gender played a role in the frequency or types of aggression.

However, Levy et al. (1996a) found that demographic differences did influence the frequency of neuropsychiatric symptoms. They found that women were more likely than men to be agitated and that the oldest patient group (i.e., 76–87 years) experienced more psychosis but less agitation than younger patients. By contrast, Cooper et al. (1990) did a retrospective, multicenter study of abnormal behaviors in 680 outpatients with probable AD and found no correlation between agitation and nonwhite race, age, duration of dementia, or education. However, they did find that male gender was associated with increased frequency of agitation and anger but not associated with other abnormal behaviors in AD.

Auchus (1997) investigated the incidence of AD in a sample of black outpatients and assessed the presence or absence of activity disturbances. These symptoms were considered present when the clinical history included ongoing disruptive agitated behaviors, ongoing disruption of the sleep–wake cycle, or both. In 33 probable AD patients, activity-level disturbances affected 12 patients (36%). Educational level did not significantly affect the activity level disturbances in the sample studied. Presence or absence of activity level symptoms was not significantly related to dementia severity as measured by the MMSE (Folstein et al. 1975) scores. However, the relatively small sample under investigation may have limited that study's power to detect such a relationship if one did exist. For the most part, age, gender, duration, and age at onset of cognitive impairment were not significantly related to particular behavioral problems, nor were they related to total numbers of behavioral problems.

The measures used to assess agitation and demographics vary across studies. Reisberg et al. (1987) did a chart review for behavioral symptoms such as delusions, agitation of a nonspecific nature, anxiety, tearful episodes, decreased appetite, mood fluctuations, and flattened affect. Aarsland et al. (1996), on the other hand, assessed patients with the Behavioral Pathology in AD rating scale (BEHAVE-AD; Reisberg et al. 1987), which assesses, among other aspects of behavioral symptoms, three aspects of aggressive behavior: verbal outbursts, physical aggression, and agitation. Levy et al. (1996b) assessed patients with the AD Assessment Scale (ADAS; Rosen et al. 1984), which primarily measures cognitive abilities but also incorporates a caregiver-rated, 10-item, noncognitive subscale for assessing neuropsychiatric symptoms. Under the rubric of agitation, this scale measures only pacing and increased motor activity. Furthermore, the patients in this study were relatively well-educated white patients with MMSE scores between 12 and 26. Because of extensive exclusion criteria, this study group had very little morbidity other than AD. A study by Cooper et al. (1990) used no specific scale for behavioral assessment. Instead, additional behaviors such as anger and wandering were examined.

In conclusion, a review of the published information shows discrepancies and similarities among investigators. The differences can possibly be explained by the varying definitions of agitation and the use of different measurement tools. Therefore, it is difficult to integrate the various findings into a comprehensive view of the correlation (if any) between agitation and demographics. Although agitation (or components of agitation) constitutes a part of the behaviors under examination in these studies, it is not possible to isolate the prevalence of agitation precisely from the presented data. Additional study is needed to determine confidently whether agitation is present at different rates in different demographic groups.

Patient Settings

Community Residents

Although various reports (Hamel et al. 1990; Reisberg et al. 1987; Swearer et al. 1988) point to the existence of behavioral problems in patients with dementia who reside outside of long-term care facilities, little systematic information exists concerning the extent and types of agitated behavior in these settings. Additionally, although existing studies of the relationship between cognitive impairment and agitation in patients with AD draw different conclusions, the relationship between cognitive impairment and agitation for AD patients residing in the community has not been studied extensively.

In a study of 183 persons with dementia of any etiology residing in the community, Ryden (1986) found more aggressive behaviors in persons with more severe cognitive impairment. In this study, 65% of the subjects were reported to have at least one form of aggression, most commonly verbal aggression. Hamel et al. (1990) reported that 57% of their community-residing patients with dementia exhibited aggressive behaviors. Verbal aggression was the most frequently reported behavior, occurring in 51% of patients, and physical aggression was reported in 34%. However, even within the category of physical aggression, the most common behavior was threatening gestures. This suggests that among community residents, the *threat* of verbal or physical aggression is more common than *actual* aggressive behavior.

Nursing Homes

Most residents of nursing homes have dementia, and many of these individuals exhibit behavioral disturbances. The National Nursing Home Survey (1977–1978) conducted by the National Center for Health Statistics (1989) reported that 66% of nursing home residents exhibited some form of behavioral disturbance. As may be expected, staffing requirements increase as the incidence of agitation increases.

Zimmer et al. (1984) surveyed skilled-nursing facilities in upstate New York and described 64.2% of the 3,456 residents as manifesting significant behavioral problems. An additional 22.6% were described as having "serious" problems that placed them at high risk for personal injury or injury to others. Malone et al. (1993) did a retrospective review of all incident reports in a 350-bed urban skilled nursing facility during a 1-year period. The type of incident was categorized as kick, bite, hit, pinch, spit, push, scratch, or other. In this study, 94 incident reports described aggressive behaviors with 48% of the aggressive behaviors occurring on the 60-bed AD unit. In fact, six residents on the AD unit accounted for 40% of all aggressive-behavior incident reports. More than 50% of these were described as one resident hitting another resident or a staff member. The study reported that 62% of the victims of aggressive behavior were other nursing home residents and 37% were nursing home employees. One victim was a visitor. Interestingly, this review showed that only two-thirds of aggressive behaviors against employees were recorded in nursing home incident reports. This suggests that, as a whole, prevalence rates for aggressive behaviors may be underreported and, therefore, underestimated in this type of patient setting.

Although aggressive behavior is a prevalent and serious behavior problem among nursing home residents, it actually occurs much less often than other forms of agitated behavior (Cohen-Mansfield et al. 1989). Cohen-Mansfield and Billig (1986) assessed the agitated behavior of 66 cognitively impaired residents in two units of a 500-bed skilled-nursing home. These units were selected because a high percentage of agitated individuals resided there. The subject's average score on the Brief Cognitive Ratings Scale (BCRS; Reisberg and Ferris 1988) indicated severely impaired cognitive functioning. A multidisciplinary team used the Cohen-Mansfield Agitation Inventory (CMAI; Cohen-Mansfield 1986), a nurse-rated questionnaire, to rate a sample of 15 men and 51 women. Results showed that specific instances of nonaggressive behaviors such as pacing and wandering, general restlessness, constant requests for attention, complaining, and negativism were the most frequently occurring agitated behaviors. Additionally, 48 of the 66 patients were considered agitated; they manifested at least one agitated behavior at a frequency of at least several times a day. A resident was classified as nonagitated if he or she exhibited agitated behaviors less than once a week. The agitated individuals did not differ from the nonagitated ones with regard to age, cognitive level, or frequency of waking up at night. However, the agitated elderly patients received more medications for agitation, had more falls, and were less continent than nonagitated elderly patients. Furthermore, Cohen-Mansfield et al. (1989) surveyed the relative frequency of the specific types of agitated behaviors manifested during a 24-hour period. The study sample included 408 (92 men and 316 women) nursing home residents with varying levels of cognitive decline. Agitation was rated using the CMAI, which rates 29 agitated behaviors on a seven-point scale of frequency. Accordingly, 93% of the residents manifested one or more agitated behaviors at least once a week. General restlessness was the most frequent agitated behavior during each of the three nursing shifts. Other frequently occurring behaviors included pacing, cursing, constant requests for attention, repeating sentences or questions, complaining, and negativism. In general, agitated behaviors were exhibited most frequently during the day, and their frequency decreased from day to evening to night. However, approximately 14% of the residents demonstrated agitated behavior during the evening.

Aronson et al. (1993) surveyed 338 residents from six nursing homes in New York City. In this study, 71 participants were men and 267 were women. Agitation was measured with the Agitation Checklist (Wild 1988) and consisted of 20 behaviors considered most problematic by family caregivers of patients with AD. The primary nursing assistant rated each behavior. This study showed that subjects with moderate and severe cognitive impairments had significantly higher agitation scores than mildly impaired subjects; as a result, they required significantly more staff supervision because of their agitation. Although research suggests a relationship between agitation and cognitive impairment in the nursing home setting, opinions differ regarding that relationship. Cohen-Mansfield et al. (1990) found a correlation between the type of agitated behavior and the degree of cognitive impairment, with aggressive behaviors being characteristic of severe cognitive dysfunction and verbal agitation being typical in less cognitively impaired subjects. Whereas Barnes et al. (1982) and Raskind et al. (1987) found agitation to be present in early stages of dementia, Reisberg et al. (1987) reported agitation to be prevalent in later stages of dementia.

Outpatient Clinics

The prevalence of agitation in outpatient settings provides a glimpse of the type of behaviors that generate help-seeking among caregivers. Reisberg et al. (1987) did a chart review of behavioral symptoms in 57 severely impaired outpatients with a diagnosis of AD. The review found that 58% of the patients had significant behavioral symptoms: agitation (48%), motor restlessness (36%), violence (30%), verbal outbursts (24%), threatening behaviors (9%), and wandering (3%).

Aarsland et al. (1996) assessed 75 outpatients with probable or possible AD. They found that 35% of the patients exhibited verbal or physical aggression. Delusional ideation was associated with verbal aggression, but physical aggression was more frequent in patients with activity disturbance and hallucinations. Mega et al. (1996) investigated the range of behavioral abnormalities in 50 outpatients with probable AD. The most common behavior was apathy, exhibited by 72% of the patients, followed by agitation in 60% and aberrant motor behavior in 38% of the patients.

In summary, the high prevalence of reported agitation in outpatient settings strongly suggests that it is one of the major reasons that persons caring for someone with dementia seek professional assistance.

Conclusions

There is growing interest in better understanding agitated behavior in persons with dementia, especially with the increasing size of the elderly population and the inevitable increase in the number of persons with AD and related disorders. The caregiving community is already experienced with the effect that dementia and its associated behavioral challenges have on resources such as finances, staff, and emotional well-being. Although there is an absence of standards-based research using uniform definitions and methodology, several studies offer a glimpse of the possible relationships between agitation and dementia.

The studies that have been done to date produced differing estimates of the prevalence of agitation in patients with dementia. Methodological issues are complex and study design varies widely. Variability in reported frequencies of agitation among studies reflects differing inclusion criteria, methodologies, and referral populations and the changing profile of behaviors as the cognitive deterioration progresses. There also is inconsistency in the reported prevalence, which may be a result of varying definitions of agitation and the type of agitation identified. Further study should yield less contradictory results if consensus can be obtained on definitions and methodologies.

Currently, it is common practice for patients with agitation to be placed in higher levels of care along with patients who are physically impaired. Is this a detrimental case mix? Is it more beneficial to place agitated residents in a separate unit? These questions, along with others, require extensive study. If it can be concluded scientifically that dementia patients in long-term care facilities exhibit symptoms of agitation at a higher rate than similar patients living in private homes, we would better understand how behavioral symptoms are modified by the care setting. This information then could be used to determine specific interventions that help reduce agitation.

References

Aarsland D, Cummings JL, Yenner G, et al: Relationship of aggressive behavior to other neuropsychiatric symptoms in patients with Alzheimer's disease. Am J Psychiatry 153:243–247, 1996

Aronson MK, Cox Post D, Guastadisegni P: Dementia, agitation, and care in the nursing home. J Am Geriatr Soc 41:507–512, 1993

Auchus AP: Demographic and clinical features of Alzheimer disease in black Americans: preliminary observations on an outpatient sample in Atlanta, Georgia. Alzheimer Dis Assoc Disord 11:38–46, 1997

Barnes R, Veith R, Okimoto J, et al: Efficacy of antipsychotic medications in behaviorally disturbed dementia patients. Am J Psychiatry 139:1170, 1982

Burns A, Jacoby R, Levy R: Psychiatric phenomena in Alzheimer's disease, IV: disorders of behaviour. Br J Psychiatry 157:86–94, 1990

Cohen D, Eisdorfer C, Gorelick P, et al: Psychopathology associated with Alzheimer's disease and related disorders. Journal of Gerontology: Medical Sciences 48:M255–M260, 1993

Cohen-Mansfield J: Agitated behaviors in the elderly, II: preliminary results in the cognitively deteriorated. J Am Geriatr Soc 34:722–727, 1986

Cohen-Mansfield J, Billig N: Agitated behaviors in the elderly, I: a conceptual review. J Am Geriatr Soc 34:711–21, 1986

Cohen-Mansfield J, Marx MS, Rosenthal AS: A description of agitation in a nursing home. Journal of Gerontology: Medical Sciences 44:M77–M84, 1989

Cohen-Mansfield J, Marx MS, Rosenthal AS: Dementia and agitation in nursing home residents: how are they related? Psychol Aging 5:3–8, 1990

Cooper JK, Mungas D, Weiler PG: Relation of cognitive status and abnormal behaviors in Alzheimer's disease. J Am Geriatr Soc 38:867–870, 1990

Eisdorfer C, Cohen D, Paveza GJ, et al: An empirical evaluation of the Global Deterioration Scale for staging Alzheimer's disease. Am J Psychiatry 149:190–194, 1992

Folstein MF, Folstein SE, McHugh PR: "Mini-Mental State": a practical method for grading the mental state of patients for the clinician. J Psychiatry Res 12:189–198, 1975

Hamel M, Gold DP, Andres D, et al: Predictors and consequences of aggressive behavior by community-based dementia patients. Gerontologist 40:206–211, 1990

Harris Y, Gorelick PB, Cohen D, et al: Psychiatric symptoms in dementia associated with stroke: a case-control analysis among predominantly African-American patients. J Natl Med Assoc 86:697–702, 1994

Levy ML, Miller BL, Cummings JL, et al: Alzheimer's disease and frontotemporal dementias: behavioral distinctions. Arch Neurol 53:687–690, 1996a

Levy ML, Cummings JL, Fairbanks LA, et al: Longitudinal assessment of symptoms of depression, agitation, and psychosis in 181 patients with Alzheimer's disease. Am J Psychiatry 153:1438–1443, 1996b

Litvan I, Mega MS, Cummings JL, et al: Neuropsychiatric aspects of progressive supranuclear palsy. Neurology 47:1184–1189, 1996

Malone ML, Thompson L, Goodwin JS: Aggressive behaviors among the institutionalized elderly. J Am Geriatr Soc 41:853–856, 1993

Mega MS, Cummings JL, Fiorello T, et al: The spectrum of behavioral changes in Alzheimer's disease. Neurology 46:130–135, 1996

Mendez MF, Selwood A, Mastri AR, et al: Pick's disease versus Alzheimer's disease: a comparison of clinical characteristics. Neurology 43:289–292, 1993

National Center for Health Statistics: The National Nursing Home Survey. Issues in Geriatric Psychiatry Adv Psychosom Med 19:113, 1989

Raskind MA, Risse SC, Lampe TH: Dementia and antipsychotic drugs. J Clin Psychiatry 48(suppl 5):16, 1987

Reisberg B, Ferris SH, et al: Brief Cognitive Rating Scale. Psychopharmacol Bull 24:629–636, 1988

Reisberg B, Borenstein J, Salob SP, et al: Behavioral symptoms in Alzheimer's disease: phenomenology and treatment. J Clin Psychiatry 48(suppl 5):9–15, 1987

Rosen WG, Mohs RC, Davis KL: A new rating scale for Alzheimer's disease. Am J Psychiatry 141:1356–1364, 1984

Ryden MB: Aggressive behavior in persons with dementia. Gerontologist 26(suppl A):228, 1986

Sultzer DL, Levin HS, Mahler ME, et al: A comparison of psychiatric symptoms in vascular dementia and Alzheimer's disease. Am J Psychiatry 150:1806–1812, 1993

Swearer JM, Drachman DA, O'Donnell BF, et al: Troublesome and disruptive behaviors in dementia. J Am Geriatr Soc 36:784–790, 1988

Teri L, Larson EB, Reifler BV: Behavioral disturbance in dementia of the Alzheimer's type. J Am Geriatr Soc 36:1–6, 1988

Teri L, Borson S, Kiyak HA, et al: Behavioral disturbance, cognitive dysfunction, and functional skill: prevalence and relationship in Alzheimer's disease. J Am Geriatr Soc 37:109, 1989

Wild K: Agitation in Alzheimer's disease: measurement and description. Dissertation Abstracts 50:3212, 1988

Zimmer JG, Watson N, Treat A: Behavioral problems among patients in skilled nursing facilities. Am J Public Health 74:1118–1121, 1984

CHAPTER 3

Neurochemistry of Agitation

Anton Porsteinsson, M.D.
Rebekah Loy, Ph.D.
Pierre N. Tariot, M.D.

Although behavioral and psychological symptoms of dementia may not signify syndromic concepts, they can nonetheless be identified, quantified, and treated (Finkel et al. 1996; Tariot and Schneider 1998). Determinants often include psychological, neurobiological, and environmental factors. In this chapter we focus on neurobiological determinants in dementia. First, we examine some of the major findings regarding neurochemistry, using Alzheimer's disease (AD) as the prototype. We then go on to identify neurochemical changes that may have specific implications for behavioral disturbances of dementia. Finally, we briefly review human and animal studies that can illuminate brain substrates responsible for some of the target behavioral symptoms associated with dementia. The goal is to provide a framework for understanding the complex array of changes that occur in particular brain neurotransmitter systems and how these changes may relate to the clinical features, treatment approaches, and prognosis of behavioral and psychological symptoms of dementia.

Neurochemical Changes in Dementia

Alzheimer's disease is a complex, multisystem disease that affects a variety of neurotransmitters and neuromodulators. Disturbances of these neurochemical systems are measured as changes in tissue levels, serum levels, or cerebrospinal fluid levels of neurotransmitters and their metabolites; changes in central nervous system (CNS) levels of biosynthetic and biodegratory enzymes; decreased CNS uptake of neurotransmitter precursors; synaptic release and reuptake of neurotransmitters; and changes in both presynaptic and postsynaptic receptor binding sites and second messenger systems.

Acetylcholine

Altered presynaptic cholinergic function in the CNS is the most extensively studied and documented neurotransmitter deficit in AD. This is manifested by structural and functional changes with neuronal loss and atrophy of the basal forebrain, especially the nucleus basalis of Meynert. There are concomitant marked reductions in the concentration of the enzyme that synthesizes acetylcholine (choline acetyltransferase) and in the vesicular acetylcholine transporter in the neocortex and hippocampus. The enzyme that degrades acetylcholine, acetylcholinesterase, is reduced in postmortem brain tissue and during life in patients with AD, as visualized by positron emission tomography, as are choline uptake and acetylcholine release in cortical slices. Despite the central cholinergic deficit, there does not appear to be a global alteration in numbers of central muscarinic acetylcholine receptors in AD; however, specific subtypes have been shown to be affected. Whereas presynaptic muscarinic cholinergic receptors degenerate along with other presynaptic cholinergic structures, postsynaptic muscarinic receptors are preserved. There are marked reductions in certain nicotinic cholinergic receptors, which are located primarily on cortical presynaptic terminals (Mesulam 1996).

Several lines of evidence link this cholinergic deficit to the cognitive losses seen in AD. In fact, the only treatment approved for AD by the U.S. Food and Drug Administration attempts to augment cholinergic neurotransmission by blocking acetylcholinesterase. Selective muscarinic and nicotinic agonists are also in development. So far, results with the muscarinic agents have been disappointing, and nicotinic agents are still in early clinical trials (Decker and Brioni 1997; Jaen and Schwarz 1997). The short-term clinical effects of cholinergic augmentation have generally been modest, possibly because of the extensive damage already suffered by the cholinergic system at the time of diagnosis, the significant age-associated decline in the uptake of circulating choline into the brain, and the possible activity of the cholinergic receptor systems.

Dopamine

Evidence of central dopaminergic dysfunction has been reported in a subgroup of patients with AD. Up to 30% of patients with AD develop extrapyramidal symptoms, and neurobiological findings indicative of such dysfunction include cytopathological changes in the substantia nigra and decreases in brain and cerebrospinal fluid dopamine metabolites and tyrosine hydroxylase activity. Dopamine D_1 receptors appear to be unaffected or modestly reduced in the neocortex and basal ganglia, but loss of D_2 receptors has been more consistently reported (Cross et al. 1984). Deficits in all of these dopaminergic indices are considerably greater when Lewy bodies are present in the neocortex and substantia nigra (Langlais et al. 1993). These dopaminergic changes likely relate to the altered motor function seen in some patients with AD, and they may relate to some aspects of cognitive dysfunction and changes in behavior.

Norepinephrine

The locus coeruleus is the major source of noradrenergic neurons innervating the CNS. Postmortem studies consistently demonstrate a decrease in the number of neurons in the locus coeruleus of patients with AD. Brain and cerebrospinal fluid norepinephrine levels in patients with AD have generally been found to be decreased compared with control subjects (Zubenko 1992), but the levels of norepinephrine's major metabolite are either unchanged or elevated (Elrod et al. 1997; Palmer et al. 1987). These data suggest increased turnover of norepinephrine and may indicate compensatory changes in response to the locus coeruleus neuronal loss. It seems likely that the main impact of altered noradrenergic function in AD is on behavior, but a role in cognition is quite possible as well.

Serotonin

Studies both in postmortem brain tissue and in the cerebrospinal fluid of living patients have suggested decreased serotonergic activity in patients with AD, corresponding to greater neuronal loss and increased numbers of neurofibrillary tangles in the brain stem raphe nuclei (Yamamoto and Hirano 1985). Concentrations of serotonin (5-HT) and its primary metabolite 5-hydroxyindoleacetic acid (5-HIAA) are decreased in some brain areas (Chen et al. 1996) and in cerebrospinal fluid (Volicer et al. 1985), with the lowest levels in the more severely affected patients. Presynaptic deficits have also been confirmed in living patients with AD, with decreased serotonin reuptake and release in brain biopsy specimens (Palmer et al. 1987) and in postmortem samples from the temporal but not the frontal cortex (Chen et al. 1996). Studies of receptor binding have found reductions in cortical 5-HT$_2$ receptors and, to a lesser extent, in 5-HT$_1$ receptors

(Cross et al. 1984). The main implication of changes in serotonergic function is likely to be altered regulation of behavior.

Excitatory Amino Acids

Glutamate is the dominant excitatory neurotransmitter in the brain. Data indicate that whereas patients with AD have a fairly severe loss of cortical, hippocampal, and striatal glutamate (Gsell et al. 1997), patients who are in the advanced stages of AD have elevated concentrations of cerebrospinal fluid glutamate and aspartate. Glutamate exerts its effects through four classes of receptors: NMDA (N-methyl-D-aspartate), AMPA (a-amino-3-hydroxy-5-methyl-4-isoxazole proprionic acid), kainate, and metabotropic receptors. Both NMDA and AMPA receptors participate in long-term potentiation (an electrophysiological model for learning and memory involving the major synaptic pathways of the hippocampus) and in excitotoxicity, both of which may be important in the pathophysiology of AD. Excitotoxicity is produced by overstimulation of NMDA and AMPA receptors, leading to excessive calcium influx into neurons as well as cell damage or death (Meldrum and Garthwaite 1990). Regional variations in the glutamate or aspartate uptake site may contribute to local excitotoxicity in AD (Scott et al. 1995). NMDA receptors as well as associated glycine and phencyclidine binding sites are reduced in the neocortex and hippocampus in patients with AD (Gsell et al. 1997). AMPA receptor binding is also reduced in the hippocampus (Dewar et al. 1990) but may be obscured by the presence of AMPA receptors in glial cells, which are increased in persons with AD (Usowicz et al. 1989). These changes in the glutaminergic system are likely to play a role in both cognition and behavior and possibly in progression of nerve cell death as well.

Gamma-Aminobutyric Acid

Gamma-aminobutyric acid (GABA) is the predominant inhibitory neurotransmitter in the neocortex and hippocampus. The evidence implicating GABAergic neurons in AD includes decreased cortical concentrations of GABA, which vary by region (Lowe et al. 1988); reduced uptake of GABA into synaptosomes; and the loss of GABA receptors in certain brain regions (Reisine et al. 1978). Benzodiazepine binding sites, which are linked to one class of GABA receptors, show no consistent alteration in patients with AD (Greenamyre and Maragos 1993). Cortical GABAergic interneurons may be lost only at a late stage of the disease. This ubiquitous neurotransmitter system undoubtedly plays a role in a wide range of brain functions.

Neuropeptides

Many neuropeptides transmitters, including cholecystokinin, neuropeptide Y, and vasoactive intestinal peptide, appear to be unchanged in patients with AD. Others, including galanin in the nucleus basalis, substance P in the neocortex, and β-endorphin in the cerebrospinal fluid, are significantly altered, but little is known of the possible clinical consequences for these changes.

Somatostatin, which is found in high concentrations in the hypothalamus, limbic system, and some cortical neurons, is reduced in the frontal and parietal cortices, superior temporal gyri, and hippocampus in postmortem tissues from patients with AD (Gabriel et al. 1996; Tamminga et al. 1987), as are somatostatin receptors. One role for somatostatin appears to be in the induction and maintenance of long-term potentiation in the hippocampus, which has been shown to be critical in the formation of memory.

Along with somatostatin, the most consistently reported neuropeptide alteration in patients with AD is the reduction in corticotropin-releasing factor (CRF) immunoreactivity, which corresponds to a loss of interneurons in the neocortex. Whereas postsynaptic CRF receptors are concomitantly upregulated (De Souza and Battaglia 1986), CRF concentrations in the cerebrospinal fluid are decreased. The reported alterations in CRF are not unique to AD, however, because similar results are reported in numerous other neurodegenerative disorders.

Implications for Behavioral Symptoms in Dementia

Reduced transmission of neuronal messages, whether associated with changes in the amount and activity of the neurotransmitter or with reduced sensitivity to it, are likely to be associated with some of the more prevalent emotional, behavioral, and cognitive disorders found in elderly patients, whether or not they coexist with dementia.

Acetylcholine

The central cholinergic deficiency in AD contributes to the memory and cognitive impairments associated with the disease as well as to the many neuropsychiatric and behavioral disorders that are prevalent. A growing body of evidence suggests that psychotic symptoms, mood disturbances, agitation, and aggression may be mediated in part by cholinergic abnormalities and that cholinergic enhancement may play a role in ameliorating the behavioral disturbances of AD (Cummings and Kaufer 1996).

Considerable evidence relates cholinergic function to neural mechanisms of emotion. The nucleus basalis of Meynert receives many afferents from the limbic system. It has been speculated that the cholinergic projections to the neocortex, hippocampus, and amygdala may play a role in communicating the emotional state of the organism to the cerebral cortex. Data concerning mood states in patients with AD and the role of cholinergic deficiency are somewhat inconsistent across studies. An imbalance between cholinergic and monoaminergic function has been postulated in the pathogenesis of mood disorders; to oversimplify, Janowsky et al. (1983) hypothesized that depression results from a cholinergic predominance and mania from an adrenergic predominance. If this were true, we would expect to see a low prevalence of mood disorders in patients with AD. In fact, although depressive symptoms are common in AD, major depression meeting full syndromal criteria is relatively uncommon and syndromal mania is rare as well (Porsteinsson et al. 1997).

In the past, concerns arose that the widespread use of acetylcholinesterase inhibitors might induce depressive symptoms in patients with AD because several studies of cholinergic agonists found them to induce depressive symptoms in some patients with AD (Davis et al. 1987; Newhouse et al. 1988). Another study, however, described mildly euphoric effects, as found with low doses of anticholinergic agents, which precipitated dysphoria and anxiety in higher doses (Sunderland et al. 1987). Recent data from controlled trials of cholinesterase inhibitors and selective muscarinic agonists failed to show either this depression-inducing effect or a consistent mood-enhancing effect (Bodick et al. 1997; Davis et al. 1992; Morris et al. 1998; Rogers and Friedhoff 1998). Taken together, the pharmacological data suggest that modulation of mood per se with these agents is inconsistent at most. Clinical experience also suggests that this is not a major concern in practice.

The role of cholinergic deficiency in the psychotic features associated with AD has been explored through pharmacological, biochemical, and structural observations. Cholinergic antagonists may provoke, and cholinesterase inhibitors and selective muscarinic agonists may ameliorate, some psychotic features in at least a portion of the patients with AD who are experiencing these symptoms. The occurrence of psychotic features in patients with AD correlates best with metabolic and perfusion abnormalities in the frontal and temporal cortex, areas that have a marked cholinergic deficit (Mentis et al. 1995; Starkstein et al. 1994; Sultzer et al. 1995) and that show similar disturbances in violent psychiatric patients (Volkow et al. 1995). Thus, cholinergic deficits may be relevant to the psychotic features exhibited by some patients with AD.

Agitation is generally more common in the later stages of AD, but it may occur at any stage of severity (Finkel et al. 1996). It has been speculated that the increase in agitation and aggression in the later stages of AD may be related to worsening cholinergic deficit (Cummings and Kaufer 1996). As is the case with psychosis, studies of brain metabolism demonstrate a relationship between agitation in AD and temporal and frontal lobe hypometabolism rather than parietal hypometabolism (Sultzer et al. 1995). Likewise, apathy or indifference, the most commonly observed behavioral disturbance in patients with AD, correlates significantly with more severe reduction in blood flow in prefrontal and anterior temporal cortices (Craig et al. 1996). Small studies with cholinergic antagonists reported exacerbation of agitation and hostility (Sunderland et al. 1987), but large clinical trials have shown that cholinesterase inhibitors and selective muscarinic agonists may reduce or exacerbate some agitated behaviors in some patients with AD (Bodick et al. 1997, Gorman et al. 1993; Kaufer et al. 1996; Morris et al. 1998). The same large trials also tend to show reduced apathy and indifference. Taken together, these findings suggest that central cholinergic deficit plays a role in behavioral disturbances in some patients with AD and that treatment interventions attempting to reduce this deficit may lead to improvement in some psychotic symptoms, apathy, and withdrawal, and may possibly have mixed effects on agitation that vary across individuals.

Dopamine

In the absence of Lewy body pathology, AD appears to be associated with only mild disruption in the dopaminergic system. When it comes to behavioral disturbances, psychosis does not appear to be associated with presynaptic dopamine function in AD (Bierer et al. 1993; Sweet et al. 1997; Zubenko 1992). There is a possible dopamine receptor gene variant associated with psychotic symptoms, but these findings are preliminary (see discussion later in chapter).

There is no clear relationship between dopamine and mood. Data for AD show hypofunction in dopamine neurotransmission or normal function in relation to depression. In patients with AD and major depression versus AD without major depression, there was greater cytopathology in the substantia nigra, but this did not translate into significant changes in dopamine levels (Zubenko 1992). Decreased cerebrospinal fluid homovanillic acid (HVA) levels were associated with greater depression in some studies but not others. A series of recent in vitro and postmortem studies, however, indicated that a relative increase in presynaptic dopaminergic transmission may be associated with aggression in patients with AD. For example, the HVA level in the cerebrospinal fluid was elevated in five patients who had histories of aggressive behavior compared with five patients without aggressive behavior (Lopez et al. 1996).

The role of dopamine in agitation is unclear. The severity of agitation and hostility in antipsychotic-free patients with AD has shown a modest correlation with plasma HVA concentrations (Sweet et al. 1997). After 15 days of antipsychotic treatment, reductions in plasma HVA correlated with improvement in these two behavioral symptoms. Sweet et al. (1998) also reported preliminary evidence that a genetic variant of the dopamine receptor was associated with psychotic symptoms and aggression in AD, but an increased level of D_2 receptors, measured by [18F] 6-fluoro-L-dopa uptake, correlated with wandering behavior in patients with AD (Meguro et al. 1997). Finally, Victoroff et al. (1996) found normal substantia nigra pars compacta (SNPC) neuron counts in 17 patients with AD and a history of aggressive behavior and reduced SNPC neuron counts in 52 patients with AD and no aggression. Neuropathological findings in the nucleus basalis and locus coeruleus did not differ between the two groups. In summary, aggressive patients with AD appear to have relatively preserved dopamine neurotransmission and may also have genetic variations in dopamine receptor subtypes.

Norepinephrine

A functional challenge study measuring cerebrospinal fluid norepinephrine in patients with AD compared with normal control subjects showed significantly greater increase in norepinephrine in the cerebrospinal fluid after a yohimbine challenge in both normal elderly subjects and those with AD compared with young control subjects. There was a tendency for the greatest response in subjects with AD (Peskind et al. 1995). A substantial portion of the subjects with AD showed behavioral arousal, agitation, and psychotic signs and symptoms, suggesting that episodically high CNS norepinephrine responsivity may contribute to behavioral disturbances in patients with dementia.

Postmortem examinations of patients with AD who had psychotic features have found relative preservation of monoaminergic nuclei; raised or relatively preserved norepinephrine levels in the substantia nigra, other subcortical areas, and the cortex; and increased densities of cortical senile plaques and neurofibrillary tangles (Zubenko 1992). Similar studies of patients with AD and major depression have shown worse neuronal loss in the locus coeruleus than in nondepressed patients with AD (Chan-Palay and Asan 1989; Zubenko 1992) as well as 10- to 20-fold decreased cortical norepinephrine levels (Zubenko 1992). These findings suggest a specific norepinephrine deficiency in patients with AD and depression and a fairly intact or increased norepinephrine function in patients with AD and psychosis. On the other hand, Hoogendijk (1998) and Hoogendijk et al. (1995) found loss of neurons in the locus coeruleus in patients with AD but no extra loss in those with comorbid depression. They also described a significant inverse relationship between the number of remaining locus coeruleus neurons and the ratio of a monoamine metabolite (3-methoxy-4-hydroxyphenylglycol [MHPG]) to norepinephrine in the frontal cortex and locus coeruleus, suggesting increased norepinephrine turnover. Although these findings are preliminary, they may eventually have implications for treatment selection.

There may also be an association between agitation and increasing cerebrospinal fluid MHPG. Along with a previously described finding of increasing cerebrospinal fluid norepinephrine and MHPG with advancing AD, it has been speculated that the increased prevalence of agitation seen in more advanced AD could be caused by norepinephrine hyperactivity. In support of this, Russo-Neustadt and Cotman (1997) and Russo-Neustadt et al. (1998) reported that whereas the tyrosine hydroxylase immunoreactive innervation of the cerebellum is preserved in aggressive patients with AD relative to nonaggressive patients, alpha-2, beta-1, and beta-2 adrenergic receptors are all increased in aggressive patients with AD relative to nonaggressive patients with AD and control subjects. The possibility that reduction in brain norepinephrine transmission may reduce disruptive, agitated, or psychotic symptoms in AD has not been explored in placebo-controlled trials, but case reports and case series suggest that beta-blockers (e.g., propranolol) may reduce rage, aggression, and agitated behaviors in some patients with AD (Shankle et al. 1995).

Serotonin

Although deficiencies in serotonergic function are fairly well established in patients with AD, they appear to be most pronounced in those with AD and behavioral disturbances (Procter et al. 1992). This finding seems consistent with both human and animal studies suggesting that serotonin (5-HT) deficiency plays a role in the pathophysiology of several psychiatric disorders such as depressive disorders, anxiety disorders, eating disorders, psychosis, and substance use disorders as well as less-well-defined neurobehavioral states such as impulsivity, suicidality, and aggression (Doudet et al. 1995; Ratey and Gordon 1993).

Depressive features associated with AD have been associated with a significant loss of 5-HT neurons in the raphe nuclei (Zubenko 1992), and

5-HT is decreased in most brain areas in depressed patients with AD (Zubenko 1992). In addition, serotonin uptake sites were reduced in post-mortem samples of frontal and temporal cortex from patients with AD with persistent depressive symptoms during life (Chen et al. 1996).

With respect to psychotic features, one study reported a decrease in 5-HT levels in the prosubiculum and a trend toward reduced levels in other cortical and subcortical regions in patients with AD and a history of psychosis compared with those with no history of psychosis (Zubenko 1992). Antipsychotic agents can interfere with serotonergic metabolism, however, and in a study that took medications into account, no significant reduction in 5-HT occurred, but there was an increase in turnover of corti-cal 5-HT in patients with AD assessed prospectively for behavioral abnor-malities (Chen et al. 1996).

With regard to agitation, a postmortem study (Palmer et al. 1987) found a relationship between decreases in cortical 5-HT and agitated behavior. Schneider et al. (1988) found that subjects with AD and significant symp-tomatic behavioral disorders, predominantly agitation and delusions, showed significantly lower platelet 3H-imipramine binding density com-pared with a control group, which may reflect central serotonin deficit. A positive correlation has been reported between anxiety and 5-HIAA levels in patients with AD. In contrast, Lawlor et al. (1995) found no significant relationship between cognitive or noncognitive measures and postmortem levels of 5-HT or 5-HIAA in the temporal cortex. Pharmacological chal-lenge paradigm studies also lend support for a relationship between al-tered serotonin function and behavioral disturbances. Patients with AD showed greater behavioral responses, including agitation and restless-ness, after administration of the selective serotonin agonist M-chlorophe-nylpiperazine (mCPP) than did a normal control group. It was speculated that a hyperresponsive serotonergic system could account for the frequent occurrence of behavioral disturbance in patients with AD (Lawlor et al. 1989). Similarly, it has been hypothesized that changes in serotonergic re-ceptors could favor the inhibition of neuronal firing, such that the thera-peutic effect of selective serotonin reuptake inhibitors on disturbances of mood and behavior in AD might result from a reduction in 5-HT_{1a}-mediated hyperpolarization.

Serotonergic enhancement through the use of serotonin reuptake in-hibitors in patients with AD has provided mixed results regarding benefi-cial behavioral effect. An older study of alaproclate, a review of controlled studies of citalopram, two recent open trials of citalopram, a controlled study of fluvoxamine, and anecdotal reports of sertraline have indicated positive effects, but an open report of fluoxetine showed no benefit (Tariot and Schneider 1998). Large controlled studies are needed to define the potential usefulness of this class of agents.

Gamma Aminobutyric Acid

Gamma aminobutyric acid has an important role in modulating different forms of anxiety, fear, phobias, and depression, and decreased GABA activity has been associated with aggression in animal studies (Kalueff and Nutt 1996). $GABA_A$ receptors, which bind benzodiazepines and are responsible for their anxiolytic effects, are concentrated in the hippocampus and extended amygdala, areas that are greatly affected in patients with AD (Tallman and Gallager 1985). Little is known about changes in the GABA neurotransmitter system in behavioral disturbances in AD, but benzodiazepines have been used successfully to treat aggressive behavior in psychotic patients (Eichelman 1990). The utility of treating behavioral symptoms with anticonvulsants such as valproate, which enhances GABA release, lends support to a role for GABA dysfunction in agitation. The mechanism of action of this and other anticonvulsants, which have also been used to stabilize manic-depressive mood swings, is likely to be complex, however, and to involve actions other than increasing GABAergic inhibition. Attempts to treat patients with AD with more selective GABA agonists did not improve cognitive function, and studies to date have not addressed behavioral changes.

Neuropeptides and Excitatory Amino Acids

The role of CRF in cognitive or behavioral disturbances in patients with dementia has not been determined. However, the putative changes deserve special attention because of the clear relevance of CRF to behavioral and physiological responses to stress and its postulated involvement in major depression and anxiety disorders (Weiss et al. 1994). Indeed, many of the seemingly diverse pharmacotherapies that have been used successfully to treat behavioral symptoms in dementia may have a common mechanism in regulating CRF because release is stimulated by norepinephrine and acetylcholine and is inhibited by GABA (Gold et al. 1988).

Several psychiatric and other neurodegenerative disorders are associated with decreased cerebrospinal fluid somatostatin concentrations (Nemeroff and Bissette 1986). Little is known about the clinical consequences of this deficiency.

The data available on other neuropeptides and excitatory amino acids in regard to behavioral disturbances in patients with AD are too limited for inclusion in this review.

A Proposed Neurobiological Basis for Agitation in Dementia

In patients with AD, behavioral symptoms usually emerge some time after cognitive impairment, suggesting that there is a secondary degenerative process in brain regions remote from the initial site of damage. A region of the forebrain known as the extended amygdala has received considerable attention as a potential substrate for many neuropsychiatric disorders and is likely to undergo later degeneration or deafferentation in AD. This region, which forms a ring around the basal ganglia and internal capsule, includes the shell of the accumbens, nucleus basalis of Meynert, central nucleus of the amygdala, and bed nucleus of the stria terminalis. Through its connections with the orbitofrontal and temporal association cortices, hippocampus, hypothalamus, and periaqueductal gray, it is ideally situated to integrate autonomic, endocrine, and somatomotor aspects of emotional and motivational states (Andreasen 1997; Heimer et al. 1997).

The extended amygdala receives a heavy dopamine innervation and contains unique dopaminergic receptors that may form the basis of agitation symptoms responsive to antipsychotic agents. It is a rich source of many of the opioid peptides and neuropeptides, including cholecystokinin, somatostatin, neurotensin, vasopressin, and oxytocin, that are disturbed in neuropsychiatric disorders. Its CRF-containing neurons are important in physiological responses to stress and are likely to be involved in depression and anxiety disorders (Nemeroff and Bissette 1986). The region also contains many androgen-sensitive neurons, which may be involved in aggressive, sexual, and asocial components of agitated behavior. In this regard, stereotactic removal of a component of the extended amygdala has been used successfully to treat patients with pathological aggressivity.

The extended amygdala is also an important source of substance P, and in both clinical and experimental studies, there is converging evidence for a role of substance P in the control of mood, affect, and behaviors such as agitation and aggression. Whereas injection of synthetic substance P fragments can elicit isolation-induced fighting in normal mice (Hall and Stewart 1984), aggression elicited by stimulating the projection from medial amygdala to ventromedial hypothalamus is blocked by substance P antagonists (Han et al. 1996). Similarly, genetic knockout of the substance P receptor eliminates both stress-induced analgesia and the aggressive response to territorial challenge in mice (DeFelipe et al. 1998). Kramer et al. (1998) recently showed that treatment with a selective substance P antagonist significantly ameliorates symptoms of depression and anxiety. Substance P is one of the earliest neurotransmitters affected in both AD and Huntington's disease, another neurodegenerative disorder with significant behavioral symptoms. Whereas substance P–containing deep cortical interneurons are lost relatively early in AD, a substance P–containing subset of cholinergic neurons of the nucleus basalis of Meynert is affected at later stages (Ang and Shul 1995; Kowall et al. 1993).

Another neuroactive molecule, nitric oxide, may also play a role in aggression associated with AD. Nitric oxide is a novel messenger molecule that acts as a retrograde signal for long-term potentiation and other forms of neuronal plasticity. Recently, genetic studies have shown that mice null for the neuronal nitric oxide synthase (nNOS) enzyme are excessively aggressive, sexually overactive, and lacking in social inhibition (Nelson et al. 1995). This behavioral phenotype is duplicated in mice treated with nNOS inhibitors (Demas et al. 1997). Nitric oxide is normally expressed in subpopulations of neurons in the frontal and entorhinal cortex, hippocampus, amygdala, and brain stem, some of which are vulnerable in AD (Thorns et al. 1998) and in dementia associated with amyotrophic lateral sclerosis (Kuljis and Schelper 1996). Although tantalizing, a well-defined role for substance P, nitric oxide, and other neurotransmitter- or second messenger–specific pathways in aggression or agitation remains to be elucidated.

Conclusions

Although our understanding of the underlying neurobiology of AD is advancing rapidly, the neurochemistry of the wide range of behavioral and psychological symptoms of AD is far less well understood. The literature draws conflicting conclusions, most likely because of methodological problems, including qualification and quantification of the behavioral substrates, and the fleeting nature of behavioral symptoms, often lasting only minutes to hours. This suggests that the neurobiological changes of behavior are dynamic and involve biochemical and structural causes rather than static structural causes alone. The course of symptomatology in AD further supports this conclusion. Whereas cognitive functioning generally declines progressively with minor fluctuations, behavioral changes frequently are of later onset, are intermittent, and are recurrent.

A better understanding of the pattern of neuronal degeneration and involvement of structures and neurotransmitter systems known to affect behavior will be fundamental in our efforts to become more successful in therapeutic interventions for behavioral and psychological signs and symptoms in patients with AD. The future of research in this area will require integration across neurobiological and clinical investigation and must capitalize on the growing information base and novel neurochemical and neuropathological approaches available to us.

References

Andreasen NC: Linking mind and brain in the study of mental illnesses: a project for a scientific psychopathology. Science 275:1586–1593, 1997

Ang LC, Shul DD: Peptidergic neurons of subcortical white matter in aging and Alzheimer's brain. Brain Res 674:329–335, 1995

Bierer LM, Knott PJ, Schmeidler JM, et al: Post-mortem examination of dopaminergic parameters in Alzheimer's disease: relationship to noncognitive symptoms. Psychiatry Res 49:211–217, 1993

Bodick NC, Offen WW, Shannon HE, et al: The selective muscarinic agonist xanomeline improves both the cognitive deficits and behavioral symptoms of Alzheimer disease. Alzheimer Dis Assoc Disord 11(suppl 4):16–22, 1997

Chan-Palay V, Asan E: Alterations in catecholamine neurons of the locus coeruleus in senile dementia of the Alzheimer type and in Parkinson's disease with and without dementia and depression. J Comp Neurol 287:373–392, 1989

Chen CP, Alder JT, Bowen DM, et al: Presynaptic serotonergic markers in community-acquired cases of Alzheimer's disease: correlations with depression and neuroleptic medication. J Neurochem 66:1592–1598, 1996

Craig AH, Cummings JL, Fairbanks L, et al: Cerebral blood flow correlates of apathy in Alzheimer disease. Arch Neurol 53:1116–1120, 1996

Cross AJ, Crow TJ, Ferrier IN, et al: Striatal dopamine receptors in Alzheimer-type dementia. Neurosci Lett 52:1–6, 1984

Cummings JL, Kaufer D: Neuropsychiatric aspects of Alzheimer's disease: the cholinergic hypothesis revisited. Neurology 47:876–883, 1996

Davis KL, Hollander E, Davidson M, et al: Induction of depression with oxotremorine in patients with Alzheimer's disease. Am J Psychiatry 144:468–471, 1987

Davis KL, Thal LJ, Gamzu ER, et al: A double-blind placebo-controlled multicenter study of tacrine for Alzheimer's disease. N Engl J Med 327:1253–1259, 1992

Decker MW, Brioni JD: Neuronal nicotinic receptor: potential treatment of Alzheimer's disease with novel cholinergic channel modulators, in Pharmacological Treatment of Alzheimer's Disease: Molecular and Neurobiological Foundations. Edited by Brioni JD, Decker M. New York, Wiley-Liss, Inc. 1997, pp 433–459

DeFelipe C, Herrero JF, O'Brien JA, et al: Altered nociception, analgesia and aggression in mice lacking the receptor for substance P. Nature 392:394–397, 1998

Demas GE, Eliasson MJ, Dawson TM, et al: Inhibition of neuronal nitric oxide synthase increases aggressive behavior in mice. Mol Med 3:610–616, 1997

De Souza EB, Battaglia G: Increased corticotropin-releasing factor receptors in rat cerebral cortex following chronic atropine treatment. Brain Res 397:401–404, 1986

Dewar D, Chalmers DT, Shand A, et al: Selective reduction of quisqualate (AMPA) receptors in Alzheimer cerebellum. Ann Neurol 28:805–810, 1990

Doudet D, Hommer D, Higley JD, et al: Cerebral glucose metabolism, CSF 5-HIAA levels, and aggressive behavior in rhesus monkeys. Am J Psychiatry 152:1782–1787, 1995

Eichelman BS: Neurochemical and psychopharmacologic aspects of aggressive behavior. Annu Rev Med 41:149–158, 1990

Elrod R, Peskind ER, DiGiacomo L, et al: Effects of Alzheimer's disease severity on cerebrospinal fluid norepinephrine concentration. Am J Psychiatry 154:25–30, 1997

Finkel SI, Costa E, Silva J, et al: Behavioral and psychological signs and symptoms of dementia: a consensus statement on current knowledge and implications for research and treatment. Int Psychogeriatr 8(suppl):497–500, 1996

Gabriel SM, Davidson M, Haroutunian V, et al: Neuropeptide deficits in schizophrenia vs. Alzheimer's disease cerebral cortex. Biol Psychiatry 39:82–91, 1996

Gold PW, Goodwin FK, Chrousos GP: Clinical and biochemical manifestations of depression. Relation to the neurobiology of stress. N Engl J Med 319:348–353, 1988

Gorman DG, Read S, Cummings JL: Cholinergic therapy of behavioral disturbances in Alzheimer's disease. Neuropsychiatry, Neuropsychology and Behavioral Neurology 6:229–234, 1993

Greenamyre JT, Maragos WF: Neurotransmitter receptors in Alzheimer disease. Cerebrovasc Brain Metab Rev 5:61–94, 1993

Gsell W, Strein I, Krause U, et al: Neurochemical abnormalities in Alzheimer's disease and Parkinson's disease: a comparative review. J Neural Transm Suppl 51:145–159, 1997

Hall ME, Stewart JM: Modulation of isolation-induced fighting by N- and C-terminal analogs of substance P: evidence for multiple recognition sites. Peptides 5:85–89, 1984

Han Y, Shaikh MB, Siegel A: Medial amygdaloid suppression of predatory attack behavior in the cat, I: role of a substance P pathway from the medial amygdala to the medial hypothalamus. Brain Res 716:59–71, 1996

Heimer L, Harlan RE, Alheid GF, et al: Substantia innominata: a notion which impedes clinical-anatomical correlations in neuropsychiatric disorders. Neuroscience 76:957–1006, 1997

Hoogendijk WJ: Do clinico-pathological correlates in depressed or agitated AD patients provide a rationale for specific pharmacotherapeutic strategies? 6th International Conference on Alzheimer's Disease and Related Disorders, Amsterdam, 1998

Hoogendijk WJ, Pool CW, Troost D, et al: Image analyser-assisted morphometry of the locus coeruleus in Alzheimer's disease, Parkinson's disease and amyotrophic lateral sclerosis. Brain 118:131–143, 1995

Jaen JC, Schwarz RD: Development of muscarinic agonists for the symptomatic treatment of Alzheimer's disease, in Pharmacological Treatment of Alzheimer's Disease: Molecular and Neurobiological Foundations. Edited by Brioni JD, Decker MW. New York, Wiley-Liss, Inc, 1997, pp 409–432

Janowsky DS, Risch SC, Gillin JC: Adrenergic-cholinergic balance and the treatment of affective disorders. Prog Neuropsychopharmacol Biol Psychiatry 7:297–307, 1983

Kalueff A, Nutt DJ: Role of GABA in memory and anxiety. Depression and Anxiety 4:100–110, 1996

Kaufer DI, Cummings JL, Christine D: Effect of tacrine on behavioral symptoms in Alzheimer's disease: an open-label study. J Geriatr Psychiatry Neurol 9:1–6, 1996

Kowall NW, Quigley BJJ, Krause JE, et al: Substance P and substance P receptor histochemistry in human neurodegenerative diseases. Regul Pept 46:174–185, 1993

Kramer MS, Cutler N, Feighner J, et al: Distinct mechanism for antidepressant activity by blockade of central substance P receptors. Science 281:1640–1645, 1998

Kuljis RO, Schelper RL: Alterations in nitrogen monoxide-synthesizing cortical neurons in amyotrophic lateral sclerosis with dementia. J Neuropsychiatry Clin Neurosci 55:25–35, 1996

Langlais PJ, Thal L, Hansen L, et al: Neurotransmitters in basal ganglia and cortex of Alzheimer's disease with and without Lewy bodies. Neurology 43:1927–1934, 1993

Lawlor BA, Sunderland T, Mellow AM, et al: Hyperresponsivity to the serotonin agonist M-chlorophenylpiperazine in Alzheimer's disease. A controlled study. Arch Gen Psychiatry 46:542–549, 1989

Lawlor BA, Ryan TM, Bierer LM, et al: Lack of association between clinical symptoms and postmortem indices of brain serotonin function in Alzheimer's disease. Biol Psychiatry 37:895–896, 1995

Lopez OL, Kaufer D, Reiter CT, et al: Relationship between CSF neurotransmitter metabolites and aggressive behavior in Alzheimer's disease. Eur J Neurol 3:153–155, 1996

Lowe SL, Francis PT, Procter AW, et al: Gamma-aminobutyric acid concentration in brain tissue at two stages of Alzheimer's disease. Brain 111:785–799, 1988

Meguro K, Yamaguchi S, Itoh M, et al: Striatal dopamine metabolism correlated with frontotemporal glucose utilization in Alzheimer's disease: a double-tracer PET study. Neurology 49:941–945, 1997

Meldrum B, Garthwaite J: Excitatory amino acid neurotoxicity and neurodegenerative disease. Trends Pharmacol Sci 11:379–387, 1990

Mentis MJ, Weinstein EA, Horwitz B, et al: Abnormal brain glucose metabolism in the delusional misidentification syndromes: a positron emission tomography study in Alzheimer disease. Biol Psychiatry 38:438–449, 1995

Mesulam MM: The systems-level organization of cholinergic innervation in the human cerebral cortex and its alterations in Alzheimer's disease. Prog Brain Res 109:285–297, 1996

Morris JC, Cyrus PA, Orazem J, et al: Metrifonate benefits cognitive, behavioral, and global function in patients with Alzheimer's disease. Neurology 50:1222–1230, 1998

Nelson RJ, Demas GE, Huang PL, et al: Behavioural abnormalities in male mice lacking neuronal nitric oxide synthase. Nature 378:383–386, 1995

Nemeroff CB, Bissette G: Neuropeptides in psychiatric disorders, in American Handbook on Psychiatry, Vol VIII. Edited by Berger P, Brodie HKH. New York, Basic Books, 1986, pp 64–110

Newhouse PA, Sunderland T, Tariot PN, et al: Intravenous nicotine in Alzheimer's disease: a pilot study. Psychopharmacology 95:171–175, 1988

Palmer AM, Wilcock GK, Esiri MM, et al: Monoaminergic innervation of the frontal and temporal lobes in Alzheimer's disease. Brain Res 401:231–238, 1987

Peskind ER, Wingerson D, Murray S, et al: Effects of Alzheimer's disease and normal aging on cerebrospinal fluid norepinephrine responses to yohimbine and clonidine. Arch Gen Psychiatry 52:774–782, 1995

Porsteinsson AP, Tariot PN, Schneider LS: Mood disturbances in Alzheimer's disease. Semin Clin Neuropsychiatry 2:265–275, 1997

Procter AW, Francis PT, Stratmann GC, et al: Serotonergic pathology is not widespread in Alzheimer patients without prominent aggressive symptoms. Neurochem Res 17:917–922, 1992

Ratey JJ, Gordon A: The psychopharmacology of aggression: toward a new day. Psychopharmacol Bull 29:65–73, 1993

Reisine TD, Yamamura HI, Bird ED, et al: Pre- and postsynaptic neurochemical alterations in Alzheimer's disease. Brain Res 159:477–481, 1978

Rogers SL, Friedhoff LT: Long-term efficacy and safety of donepezil in the treatment of Alzheimer's disease: an interim analysis of the results of a US multicentre open label extension study. Eur Neuropsychopharmacol 8:67–75, 1998

Russo-Neustadt A, Cotman CW: Adrenergic receptors in Alzheimer's disease brain: selective increases in the cerebella of aggressive patients. J Neurosci 17:5573–5580, 1997

Russo-Neustadt A, Zomorodian TJ, Cotman CW: Preserved cerebellar tyrosine hydroxylase-immunoreactive neuronal fibers in a behaviorally aggressive subgroup of Alzheimer's disease patients. Neuroscience 87:55–61, 1998

Schneider LS, Severson JA, Chui HC, et al: Platelet tritiated imipramine binding and MAO activity in Alzheimer's disease patients with agitation and delusions. Psychiatry Res 25:311–322, 1988

Scott HL, Tannenberg AE, Dodd PR: Variant forms of neuronal glutamate transporter sites in Alzheimer's disease cerebral cortex. J Neurochem 64:2193–2202, 1995

Shankle WR, Nielson KA, Cotman CW: Low-dose propranolol reduces aggression and agitation resembling that associated with orbitofrontal dysfunction in elderly demented patients. Alzheimer Dis Assoc Disord 9:233–237, 1995

Starkstein SE, Vazquez S, Petracca G, et al: A SPECT study of delusions in Alzheimer's disease. Neurology 44:2055–2059, 1994

Sultzer DL, Mahler ME, Mandelkern MA, et al: The relationship between psychiatric symptoms and regional cortical metabolism in Alzheimer's disease. J Neuropsychiatry Clin Neurosci 7:476–484, 1995

Sunderland T, Tariot PN, Cohen RM, et al: Anticholinergic sensitivity in patients with dementia of the Alzheimer type and age-matched controls. A dose-response study. Arch Gen Psychiatry 44:418–426, 1987

Sweet RA, Pollock BG, Mulsant BH, et al: Association of plasma homovanillic acid with behavioral symptoms in patients diagnosed with dementia: a preliminary report. Biol Psychiatry 42:1016–1023, 1997

Sweet RA, Nimgaonkar VL, Kamboh MI, et al: Dopamine receptor genetic variation, psychosis, and aggression in Alzheimer disease. Arch Neurol 55:1335–1340, 1998

Tallman JF, Gallager DW: The GABA-ergic system: a locus of benzodiazepine action (review). Annu Rev Neurosci 8:21–44, 1985

Tamminga CA, Foster NL, Fedio P, et al: Alzheimer's disease: low cerebral somatostatin levels correlate with impaired cognitive function and cortical metabolism. Neurology 37:161–165, 1987

Tariot PN, Schneider LS: Nonneuroleptic treatment of complications of dementia: applying clinical research to practice, in Geriatric Psychopharmacology. Edited by Nelson JC. New York, Marcel Dekker, 1998, pp 427–453

Thorns V, Hansen L, Masliah E: nNOS expressing neurons in the entorhinal cortex and hippocampus are affected in patients with Alzheimer's disease. Exp Neurol 150:14–20, 1998

Usowicz MM, Gallo V, Cull-Candy SG: Multiple conductance channels in type-2 cerebellar astrocytes activated by excitatory amino acids. Nature 339:380–383, 1989

Victoroff J, Zarow C, Mack WJ, et al: Physical aggression is associated with preservation of substantia nigra pars compacta in Alzheimer disease. Arch Neurol 53:428–434, 1996

Volicer L, Direnfeld LK, Freedman M, et al: Serotonin and 5-hydroxyindoleacetic acid in CSF: difference in Parkinson's disease and dementia of the Alzheimer's type. Arch Neurol 42:127–129, 1985

Volkow ND, Tancredi LR, Grant C, et al: Brain glucose metabolism in violent psychiatric patients: a preliminary study. Psychiatry Res 61:243–253, 1995

Weiss JM, Stout JC, Aaron MF, et al: Depression and anxiety: role of the locus coeruleus and corticotropin-releasing factor. Brain Res Bull 35:561–572, 1994

Yamamoto T, Hirano A: Nucleus raphe dorsalis in Alzheimer's disease: neurofibrillary tangles and loss of large neurons. Ann Neurol 17:573–577, 1985

Zubenko GS: Biological correlates of clinical heterogeneity in primary dementia. Neuropsychopharmacology 6:77–93, 1992

CHAPTER 4

Use of Behavioral Assessment Scales for Evaluating Agitation in Dementia

Daryl L. Bohac, Ph.D.
Dennis P. McNeilly, Psy.D.
David G. Folks, M.D.

The case reported by Alzheimer in 1907 provided a classic description of the psychopathology or noncognitive behavioral disturbances that accompanied his patient's dementia. Psychopathology rapidly faded as the primary focus in dementia, and memory loss and other cognitive changes became the major clinical focus along with the neuropathological correlates of dementia. In the 1980s, psychopathology resurfaced as a major focus of dementia research. This was evidenced by the emergence of instruments to assess agitation, delusions, hallucinations, apathy, sleep disturbance, and other signs and symptoms associated with dementia. Some of these instruments chose to emphasize different aspects of symptoms targeted for interventions—that is, some instruments focused on the frequency of symptoms, and others focused on the severity. One of the most recent scales assesses both the frequency and the severity of symptoms, along with caregiver distress that might be associated with each symptom. This issue of caregiver burden merits attention because the behavioral symptoms associated with dementia, in particular agitation and psychosis, are significant sources of stress for family members, residential care facility staff, and hospital staff.

Agitation-Specific Rating Scales

Most rating scales designed for dementia have a broad focus that allows for ratings of various domains of functions, either through direct observation or by caregiver interviews. For example, the Brief Psychiatric Rating Scale (BPRS; Overall and Gorham 1962) is commonly used to examine a broad range of behaviors, including agitation. This instrument has three-item subscales for hostility (agitation), thought disturbances (psychosis), depression, and withdrawal (apathy). Other multidimensional instruments commonly used include the Comprehensive Psychopathological Rating Scale (Bucht and Adolfsson 1983); the Alzheimer's Disease Assessment Scale, Noncognitive Subscale (Rosen et al. 1984); and the Global Deterioration Scale (Reisberg et al. 1982). (A full description of these instruments is beyond the scope of this chapter.) On the other hand, some rating scales focus specifically on the assessment of agitation.

Of the rating scales that have a specific focus on agitation, the Cohen-Mansfield Agitation Inventory (CMAI; Cohen-Mansfield et al. 1989) is perhaps the best known. The items of the CMAI were developed by interviewing nursing home staff members and reviewing the literature. Examples of item content contained in the original 29-item version of the CMAI are presented in Table 4–1. Each item is rated on a seven-point scale ranging from "never" to "several times per hour" and is self-administered by the caregiver or completed in an interview format with the caregiver. In either format, the caregiver estimates the frequency of the behaviors over the past 2 weeks.

Since the inception of the CMAI, the scale's authors have created a 14-item short form, each rated on a five-point scale of frequency. They have also developed a community form with 37 items. The items have been grouped into three areas representing physically aggressive behaviors, physically nonaggressive behaviors, and verbally agitated behaviors (Finkel et al. 1993). Meanwhile, Cohen-Mansfield (1996) has suggested that four subtypes of agitation can be identified with the CMAI: physically nonaggressive behaviors, physically aggressive behaviors, verbally nonaggressive behaviors, and verbally aggressive behaviors. The CMAI has been found to have high internal consistency and reliability, but interrater variability was high (Finkel et al. 1992). Miller et al. (1995) also found the CMAI to be internally consistent and noted significantly higher interrater reliability than previously observed.

Citing time restrictions on caregivers of nursing home residents, Finkel et al. (1993) derived a 10-item Brief Agitation Rating Scale (BARS)

Table 4–1. Behaviors rated on the Cohen-Mansfield Agitation Inventory

Physically aggressive	Physically nonaggressive	Verbally agitated
Hitting	Pacing/wandering	Screaming
Kicking	Inappropriate dress/	Cursing
Grabbing	disrobing	Verbal sexual advances
Pushing	Trying to get to a different	Repetitive questions
Throwing things	place	Strange noises
Biting	Intentional falling	Complaining
Scratching	Hiding things	Negativism
Spitting	Hoarding things	Constant unwanted
Destroying property	Repetitious mannerisms	requests for attention or
Hurting self or others	General restlessness	help
Physical sexual	Handling things	
advance	inappropriately	
	Eating/drinking	
	inappropriate substances	

from the 29-item CMAI. Using a three-step selection criteria (i.e., item to total score correlations across shifts; interrater correlations; and representation of items from the dimensions of physically aggressive behaviors, physically nonaggressive behaviors, and verbally agitated behaviors), the following items were selected for inclusion in the BARS: hitting, grabbing, pushing, pacing or wandering, performing repetitious mannerisms, acting restless, screaming, saying repetitive sentences or asking repetitive questions, making strange noises, and complaining. The BARS accounted for approximately 90% of the total variance of the total score on the CMAI across the day, evening, and night shifts of the nursing home ($r = 0.95$, 0.94, and 0.95, respectively). This suggests that the BARS may be an adequate screening instrument in nursing home settings, where there is often a need for quick and effective assessment of behavioral disturbances.

Another relatively brief rating scale for agitation was developed out of the perceived need for a rating scale that did not require assessment of specific behaviors over several days. The Pittsburgh Agitation Scale (PAS; Rosen et al. 1994) is completed based on direct observations of the patient. It purports to measure the severity of agitation, whereas the CMAI and BARS measure the frequency. On a scale of 0 to 4, the PAS rates the severity of agitation in four general behavior groups: aberrant vocalization, motor agitation, aggressiveness, and resisting care. The authors evaluated their instrument in an acute-care psychogeriatric unit and a chronic-care nursing facility. They determined that the PAS had adequate interrater reliability in either setting. Validity in the acute-care setting was determined by the need for restraints, either physical or chemical. Patients with lower PAS scores required significantly fewer interventions than patients scoring higher on the PAS. Validity in the nursing home setting was established by comparing PAS scores with real-time microcomputer monitoring scores. Significant correlations were obtained for Aberrant Vocalization, Motor Agitation, and Aggressiveness scores.

Another instrument with a specific focus on agitation is the Overt Aggression Scale (OAS; Silver and Yudofsky 1991; Yudofsky et al. 1986). However, in this case, the focus is on the frequency of global aggressiveness. This scale allows weighted scoring of verbal aggression, physical aggression against self, physical aggression against objects, and physical aggression against self or others. The scale provides an objective picture of aggressive behavior over time through weekly assessments. The OAS also allows evaluation of response to interventions.

Subsequently, Yudofsky et al. (1997) developed the Overt Agitation Severity Scale (OASS), which focuses on the severity of agitation, including aggressiveness. This scale was developed to define and objectively rate the severity of agitation. The OASS confines its ratings exclusively to observable behavioral manifestations of agitation in terms of frequency and severity based on one 15-minute observation period. The difference between the OASS and the CMAI is that the latter is a retrospective rating that uses data over 2 weeks from the domains of agitation, aggressiveness, and other problem behaviors. The OASS focuses on objectifiable verbalizations and upper- and lower-body motor behaviors. Thus, the OASS is sensitive in rating agitation severity during agitated and nonagitated periods. This may be especially useful in evaluating the effects of medication on agitation.

A scale that measures the global severity of agitation in dementia has been accepted by the U.S. Food and Drug Administration (FDA) for registering indications for the treatment of agitation. This scale is the Excited component (EC) from the Positive and Negative Symptom Scale (PANSS) developed by Kay et al. (1987) and is referred to as the PANSS-EC. The FDA accepted this instrument for indication registration on the basis of the scale's demonstrated reliability and validity in rating severity of agitation across three distinct clinical populations: schizophrenia, bipolar mania, and three subtypes of dementia (Alzheimer's disease, ischemic vascular, and mixed Alzheimer's/ischemic vascular).

The PANSS-EC consists of five items: Poor Impulse Control, Tension, Hostility, Uncooperativeness, and Excitement. Each item has associated descriptors and is rated on a scale of 1 (absence of any symptom) to 7 (extremely severe symptoms). The total score can range from 5 to 25 and a score of less than 14 indicates the absence of moderate to severe agitation. The PANSS-EC is very simple to use clinically and its sensitivity to changes induced by placebo, haloperidol, lorazepam, and olanzapine has been established. Limitations of the scale include its lack of behavioral specificity, because it provides only a global rating of agitation—that is, it does not identify individual problem behaviors (e.g., hitting, biting, spitting) or the impact of treatment interventions on specific behaviors.

Of the instruments reviewed here, the CMAI is the most widely used agitation-specific rating scale. It is used in clinical trials for Alzheimer's disease (AD) and has been described as being a potentially useful tool in assessing the effects of cognitive enhancers and other types of psychotropic drugs on behavior in patients with dementia (Koss et al. 1997). However, the CMAI has some noteworthy limitations. The length of the original version may create a time burden on staff caregivers in nursing home settings. The advent of the 14-item short form by the authors as well as the BARS are important adaptations of the CMAI, making it more likely that systematic assessment of treatment interventions will occur. The variability in interrater correlations obtained in the various studies of the CMAI point out the need for adequate training of the staff members who will be completing the rating scale. As a result, additional training may impose greater time restraints on already busy caregivers. Finally, as noted by Ferris and Mackell (1997), the CMAI does not address the impact of agitation on caregivers.

In contrast to the CMAI, and to a lesser extent the BARS, the PAS offers an alternative approach to the specific assessment of agitation. Its emphasis on direct observation reduces reliance on the use of chart notes or other sources of secondhand information when completing the scale. According to its authors, the scale can be completed in approximately 1 minute, and it can be used reliably by staff with minimal prior instruction (Rosen et al. 1994). However, specific behaviors are not assessed with the PAS, and other sources would have to be used to obtain such information. This seems a significant shortcoming because interventions are often targeted at specific symptoms. In addition, the authors note that the PAS is environment specific—that is, a score obtained in an acute-care setting may not generalize to other settings. This scale may be most appropriate when attempting to determine the level of overall agitation in a specific environment. If more specific information about the behaviors of concern is required, clinicians and researchers may be better served with the CMAI.

Broadly Focused Rating Scales of Noncognitive Disturbances

One of the earliest broad-focus instruments to emerge was the Behavioral Pathology in Alzheimer's Disease rating scale (BEHAVE-AD; Reisberg et al. 1987). Conducting retrospective chart reviews on 55 patients with AD, these authors noted that the two most common symptoms reported were delusions of theft and agitation. They also observed that of the various instruments available at that time, none was appropriate for assessing "the magnitude of pharmacologically remediable behavioral symptomology [*sic*] in the Alzheimer's patient" (p. 5). In response to this identified need, the authors developed the BEHAVE-AD, which they designed to 1) specifically measure characteristic behavioral symptoms that commonly occur in AD; 2) be independent of the cognitive symptomatology of AD; 3) reflect the concerns identified by caregivers; and 4) target behaviors that were thought to be remediable through pharmacological or other interventions. Table 4–2 lists the domains assessed by the 25-item BEHAVE-AD.

Each of the areas assessed by the BEHAVE-AD uses multiple items to evaluate the severity of the behavioral disturbance. Agitation is assessed by two groups of items under the general headings of "Activity Disturbances" and "Aggressivity." For the former, three items evaluate wandering, purposeless behavior, and inappropriate behavior. Under the latter heading, three items tap into verbal outbursts, physical threats or violence, and agitation other than the previous two areas. Each item is rated on a four-point scale, with zero indicating the behavior is not present and higher scores reflecting a more severe disturbance. For example, the assessor is asked to determine whether agitation is present, and if so, whether there is an emotional component or an emotional and physical component, with the latter area being rated as representing the most severe element of nonspecific agitation.

Mack and Patterson (1994) investigated the usefulness of the BEHAVE-AD along with the Cornell Scale for Depression (Alexopoulos et al. 1988) and the BPRS. One of the most useful aspects of this study was its discussion of the problems encountered by the raters when administering the three rating scales. One problem with the BEHAVE-AD concerned the clarity of item meaning. For example, a group of items are clustered under the general heading of "Aggressivity." The first (item 16), is concerned with verbal outbursts, the second (item 17) is labeled "physical threats and/or violence," and the third (item 18) is "agitation (other than above)." Although items 16 and 17 are adequately specific, the third item of the group appears to be a catch-all item that may introduce vagueness rather

Table 4–2. Noncognitive behavioral domains assessed by each broadly focused instrument

Instrument	Domain
BEHAVE-AD	Paranoid and delusional ideation
	Hallucinations
	Activity disturbances
	Aggressivity
	Diurnal rhythm disturbance
	Affective disturbances
	Anxieties and phobias
	Global rating of distress/dangerousness
CERAD BRSD	Psychotic symptoms
	Depressive symptoms
	Behavioral dysregulation
	Irritability/agitation
	Inertia
	Vegetative
COBRA	Assaultive/aggressive
	Ideas/personality
	Mechanical/motor
	Vegetative
NPI	Delusions
	Hallucinations
	Agitation/aggression
	Dysphoria
	Anxiety
	Euphoria
	Apathy
	Disinhibition
	Irritability/lability
	Aberrant motor behavior
	Nighttime behavior[a]
	Appetite/eating changes[a]

Note. BEHAVE-AD = Behavioral Pathology in Alzheimer's Disease; CERAD BRSD = Consortium to Establish a Registry for Alzheimer's Disease Behavior Rating Scale for Dementia; COBRA = Caretaker Obstreperous-Behavior Rating Assessment; NPI = Neuropsychiatric Inventory.
[a]Found only on the nursing home version of the NPI.

than behavioral specificity. Also of concern to the raters were the differing behaviors on which severity judgments were sometimes based. As noted by Mack and Patterson (1994), "the presence of violence in association with a particular behavior was used to differentiate severity level in six of 25 items, and there was also another item specifically related to violence" (p. 115). Finally, many caregivers who served as informants in this study also required additional explanation when completing the rating scale. Despite these concerns, several studies have demonstrated the reliability and validity of the BEHAVE-AD (Mack and Patterson 1994; Patterson et al. 1990; Sclan et al. 1996).

Although the BEHAVE-AD assesses the severity of agitation and other behavioral disturbances in patients with dementia, Tariot et al. (1995) chose to emphasize frequency ratings of the behavior, citing the difficulty in reliably determining the severity with which the behavior of concern occurs. Tariot et al. (1995), from the behavioral pathology committee of the Consortium to Establish a Registry for Alzheimer's Disease (CERAD), developed the Behavior Rating Scale for Dementia (BRSD). Borrowing from many sources, including the BEHAVE-AD, the Columbia University Scale for Psychopathology in Alzheimer's Disease (Devanand et al. 1992), and the Cornell Scale for Depression in Dementia, they developed a 51-item scale. A large-scale, multicenter study then followed in which nearly 600 persons with AD were used to produce the 46-item version of the BRSD (Mack and Patterson 1996). These items were subjected to principal-axis factor analysis using Varimax rotation, which yielded six interpretable factors labeled psychotic symptoms, depressive symptoms, behavioral dysregulation, irritability/agitation, inertia, and vegetative, respectively. Normative information has been developed for the subscales based on these six interpretable factors. A 17-item short form has also been developed. All items are rated on a scale ranging from 0 ("has not occurred since illness began") to 4 ("16 days or more in past month"). In addition, each item can be rated as having occurred before the 1-month assessment window or can be scored as "unable to rate" if the informant does not have any knowledge about the behavior being rated.

In both the original study of the BRSD (Tariot et al. 1995) and the subsequent revision, the BRSD proved to have robust interrater reliability. This is, in part, because of the comprehensive instructions and training provided to the raters in these studies. Patterson et al. (1997) investigated the test–retest reliability and sensitivity to change of the BRSD and found its 1-month test–retest reliability to be satisfactory. They also found that the BRSD was effective at discriminating healthy elderly persons from persons with AD. Although not finding the BRSD sensitive to 12-month interval changes, the authors argued that the variability in noncognitive changes, as some symptoms disappear and others appear, may actually lead to stability of total BRSD scores. For this reason, it is important to examine the subscale scores when evaluating change across longer intervals rather than focusing exclusively on the total score when using the BRSD.

One of the earliest attempts at systematically evaluating both the frequency and the severity of noncognitive behavioral disturbance in dementia was by Drachman et al. (1992), who developed the Caretaker Obstreperous-Behavior Rating Assessment (COBRA) scale for use by family or professional caregivers. It was designed to classify behaviors into four categories: aggressive/assaultive, mechanical/motor, ideas/personality, and vegetative, with 30 specific behaviors identified. The frequency of each target behavior is from 0 (absent in the past 3 months) to 4 (a behavior that has occurred daily or more often). The severity of the behavior is similarly rated, with a range from 0 (no appreciable disruptive effect) to 4 (behavior judged to present a significant danger). Twelve summary scores are then generated from the frequency and severity ratings of the COBRA. They are designed to reflect which behavioral categories are present, how many different behaviors are present, how severely disruptive the behaviors are, and how frequently the behaviors occur. The initial study by Drachman et al. (1992) found COBRA to have good test–retest reliability for 11 of the 12 summary scores. Only a modest test–retest correlation for the highest frequency score, $r=0.44$, was found. Interrater reliability ranged from .99 to .73 for 8 of the 12 summary scores, whereas 4 of the scores had modest correlations of .68 or less. Of note, the latter results were found with the vegetative disorders scores and the total number of disordered ideas or personality behaviors.

One of the latest instruments to emerge that assesses behavioral disturbance in AD is the Neuropsychiatric Inventory (NPI; Cummings et al. 1994). The NPI measures both the frequency and severity of behavioral disturbance as well as intensity of distress experienced by caregivers for each domain. In their initial study, Cummings et al. (1994) demonstrated content and concurrent validity as well as interrater, test–retest, and internal consistency reliability of the NPI. The indices of reliability and concurrent validity were based on behavioral information provided by family caregivers of outpatients attending a university or Veterans Affairs dementia clinic or of patients who were receiving stable doses of medication in a clinical trial program. None of the patients in the initial study were institutionalized in nursing care facilities or other structured residential programs. Thus, with the exception of the content validity data, the initial psychometric findings may limit the use of the NPI to relatively high-functioning patients with dementia until additional normative data for other populations is available.

Since the introduction of the original NPI, Cummings (personal communication, May 1, 1996) has developed a Nursing Home version (NPI/NH). The NPI/NH differs from the NPI in that it reflects different places of residence and different informant sources. The NPI/NH recognizes professional caregivers such as nurses and nursing assistants as informants and asks about level of occupational distress rather than level of emotional distress. The NPI and NPI/NH both use a screen and metric approach to the assessment of behavioral disturbance. For example, when asked about delusions, the informant is asked if the patient has beliefs that are known not to be true and is then given examples of a delusional belief. If the informant answers no, then the rater proceeds to the next screening question. However, if the informant answers yes, then a series of questions are asked to more fully illuminate the nature of the patient's delusional beliefs and to better ascertain the frequency and severity of the behavioral disturbance.

All of the broadly focused rating scales of noncognitive disturbance in dementia reviewed in this chapter have measures of agitation subsumed with their respective item content. One possible disadvantage is that agitation measures may be spread across more than one subscale of the instrument. If the CMAI is used as the standard by which to judge the groupings of items on these broadly based scales, then the BEHAVE-AD has two subscales, Activity Disturbances and Aggressivity, that contain items similar to those found on the CMAI. Similarly, the CERAD BRSD uses two content areas, Behavioral Dysregulation and Irritability/Agitation. The COBRA also uses two content areas (i.e., Assaultive/Aggressive and Mechanical/Motor), as does the NPI (i.e., Agitation and Aberrant Motor Behavior), that capture the same or similar items found on the CMAI. However, this may allow for greater specificity of type of agitation being expressed by the person with dementia.

The use of informant-based ratings of agitation has received considerable attention. One issue is who should be an informant for these ratings. The CERAD BRSD manual states:

> The informant, ideally, should be the primary caregiver of the subject of the interview and in daily contact with the subject. At a minimum the informant should have been in face-to-face contact with the subject on a regular basis at least two days per week during the month prior to the interview. (Mack and Patterson 1996, p. 3)

This appears to be a reasonable guideline to follow. Although achieving the ideal of a caregiver in daily contact may not be possible, lowering the threshold from 2 days of contact per week, as suggested by Mack and Patterson (1996), runs the risk of invalid information that may in turn lead to erroneous conclusions about the patient.

Concerns have also been raised about the reliability of information obtained from family caregivers of persons with dementia. Caregivers are at risk for burnout and depression associated with the demands of caring for a chronically ill patient. If, for example, the severity of the patient's behavioral symptoms is exaggerated, then there is the risk for inappropriate treatment of the patient. It may be that the caregiver is the one who requires treatment. In other cases, it is the person with dementia who requires treatment, or it may be both the caregiver and the person with dementia who need treatment. Using multiple sources of information can help to minimize the possibility of erroneous information, whether is it more than one informant or serial assessment using the same informant.

Perhaps the most important issue to consider when using any assessment device is the degree of familiarity the rater has with the instrument being used. Burgio's (1996) caveats about the importance of direct observation notwithstanding, mastery of the instrument before it is used in either clinical or research settings is critical to ensuring the reliability and validity of the rating scores. To this end, several of the instruments (e.g., NPI, COBRA) offer videotape training, and others (e.g., NPI, CMAI, BRSD) provide comprehensive instructions. In the latter category, the BRSD offers the most comprehensive set of instructions. Understanding the normative base of the instrument is part of having familiarity with the instrument. Again, the BRSD offers comprehensive normative information derived from the CERAD instrumentation studies. The available literature on the NPI also provides normative information but is limited to date. The distinct advantage with the BRSD scale is that its information is contained in a single source rather than a series of journal articles, as is the case with the other instruments.

Conclusions

Although the list of behavioral scales reviewed in this chapter is not exhaustive, it is representative of the scales available to clinicians and researchers alike. Each behavioral scale has relative strengths and weaknesses, but all of the full-length versions of the instruments have adequate reliability and validity. This is important when attempting to evaluate the efficacy of interventions targeting agitation in patients with dementia. The agitation-specific screening instruments, the BARS and PAS, should be used with some caution if comprehensive profiles of agitation are being sought. Screening instruments typically have adequate sensitivity, but they may have relatively limited specificity for the behaviors of concern. With limited specificity, one may not be able to adequately assess the efficacy of the intervention used. The systematic use of behavioral ratings is often critical in the demonstration of efficacy to family and professional caregivers alike. This is particularly true if the intervention has a behavioral component to it, the results of which are not often immediately apparent. Finally, it is necessary for both clinicians and researchers to fully evaluate the behavioral instrument themselves. Failure to understand the psychometric properties of the instruments and how well they fit with the intended purpose are sure ways of reaching disappointing, if not misleading, conclusions about interventions in the treatment of agitation in dementia.

References

Alexopoulos GS, Abrams RC, Young RC, et al: Cornell Scale for Depression in dementia. Biol Psychiatry 23:271–284, 1988

Bucht G, Adolfsson R: The comprehensive psychopathological rating scale in patients with dementia of Alzheimer type and multi-infarct dementia. Acta Psychiatr Scand 68:263–270, 1983

Burgio L: Direct observation of behavioral disturbances of dementia and their environmental context. Int Psychogeriatr 8(suppl 3):343–346, 1996

Cohen-Mansfield J: Conceptualization of agitation: results based on the Cohen-Mansfield Agitation Inventory and the Agitation Behavior Mapping Instrument. Int Psychogeriatr 8(suppl 3):309–315, 1996

Cohen-Mansfield J, Marx MS, Rosenthal AS: A description of agitation in a nursing home. Journal of Gerontology: Medical Sciences 44:M77–M84, 1989

Cummings JL, Mega M, Gray K, et al: The Neuropsychiatric Inventory: comprehensive assessment of psychopathology in dementia. Neurology 44:2308–3214, 1994

Devanand DP, Miller L, Richards M, et al: The Columbia University Scale for Psychopathology in Alzheimer's Disease. Arch Neurol 49:371–376, 1992

Drachman DA, Swearer JM, O'Donnell BF, et al: The Caretaker Obstreperous-Behavior Rating Assessment (COBRA) scale. J Am Geriatr Soc 40:463–480, 1992

Ferris SH, Mackell JA: Behavioral outcomes in clinical trials for Alzheimer disease. Alzheimer Dis Assoc Disord 11(suppl)4:10–15, 1997

Finkel SI, Lyons, JS, Anderson RL: Reliability and validity of the Cohen-Mansfield Agitation Inventory in institutionalized elderly. Int J Geriatr Psychiatry 7:487–490, 1992

Finkel SI, Lyons, JS, Anderson RL: A brief agitation rating scale (BARS) for nursing home elderly. J Am Geriatr Soc 41:50–52, 1993

Kay SR, Fishbein A, Opler LA: The positive and negative syndrome scale (PANSS) for schizophrenia. Schizophr Bull 13:261-276, 1987

Koss E, Weiner M, Ernesto C, et al: Assessing patterns of agitation in Alzheimer's disease patients with the Cohen-Mansfield Agitation Inventory: the Alzheimer's disease cooperative study. Alzheimer Dis Assoc Disord 11(suppl 2):45–50, 1997

Mack JL, Patterson MB: The evaluation of behavioral disturbances in Alzheimer's disease: the utility of three rating scales. J Geriatr Psychiatry Neurol 7:101–117, 1994

Mack JL, Patterson MB: Manual: CERAD Behavior Rating Scale for Dementia. Cleveland, OH, Consortium to Establish a Registry for Alzheimer's Disease, 1996

Miller RJ, Snowdon J, Vaughan R: The use of the Cohen-Mansfield Agitation Inventory in the assessment of behavioral disorders in nursing homes. J Am Geriatr Soc 43:546–549, 1995

Overall JE, Gorham DR: Introduction: The Brief Psychiatric Rating Scale. Psychol Rep 10:799–812, 1962

Patterson MB, Schnell, AH, Martin, RJ, et al: Assessment of behavioral and affective symptoms in Alzheimer's disease. J Geriatr Psychiatry Neurol 3:21–30, 1990

Patterson MB, Mack JL, Mackell, JA, et al: A longitudinal study of behavioral pathology across five levels of dementia severity in Alzheimer's disease: the CERAD Behavior Rating Scale for Dementia. Alzheimer Dis Assoc Disord 11(suppl 2):40–44, 1997

Reisberg B, Ferris SH, DeLeon MH, et al: The Global Deterioration Scale for assessment of primary degenerative dementia. Am J Psychiatry 139:1136–1139, 1982

Reisberg B, Borenstein J, Franssen E, et al: BEHAVE-AD: a clinical rating scale for the assessment of pharmacologically remedial behavioral symptomology in Alzheimer's disease, in Alzheimer's Disease. Edited by Altman HJ. New York, Plenum, 1987

Rosen J, Burgio L, Kollar M, et al: The Pittsburgh Agitation Scale: a user friendly instrument for rating agitation in dementia patients. Am J Geriatr Psychiatry 2:52–59, 1994

Rosen WG, Mohs RC, Davis KL: A new rating scale for Alzheimer's disease. Am J Psychiatry 141:1356–1364, 1984

Sclan SG, Saillon A, Franssen E, et al: The Behavioral Pathology in Alzheimer's Disease Rating Scale (BEHAVE-AD): reliability and analysis of symptom category scores. Int J Geriatr Psychiatry 11:819–830, 1996

Silver JM, Yudofsky SC: The Overt Aggression Scale: overview and guiding principles. J Neuropsychiatry Clin Neurosci 3(suppl 1):22–29, 1991

Tariot PN, Mack JL, Patterson MB, et al: The Behavior Rating Scale for Dementia of the Consortium to Establish a Registry for Alzheimer's Disease. Am J Psychiatry 152:1349–1357, 1995

Yudofsky SC, Silver JM, Jackson W, et al: The Overt Aggression Scale for the objective rating of verbal and physical aggression. Am J Psychiatry 143:35–39, 1986

Yudofsky SC, Kopecky HJ, Kunik ME, et al: The Overt Agitation Severity Scale for the objective rating of agitation. J Neuropsychiatry Clin Neurosci 9:541–548, 1997

CHAPTER 5

Differential Diagnosis of Agitation in Dementia

Delirium, Depression, Psychosis, and Anxiety

Joy Webster, M.D., M.P.H.
George T. Grossberg, M.D.

The noncognitive abnormalities that most commonly accompany Alzheimer's disease (AD) are behavioral abnormalities, mood disorders, and psychotic phenomena. Behavioral problems are a well-recognized complication of the progression of dementia. The most frequently reported behavioral problem is agitation, and the most frequently noted examples of agitation are restlessness; wandering; pacing; hitting or kicking; disrobing; screaming; repetitive unwarranted questions, requests, or statements; and verbal aggression. Agitated behavior is a multidimensional, complex concept in terms of assessment and intervention (Roper et al. 1991). Agitation is a highly heterogeneous syndrome, both phenomenologically and etiologically. During evaluation of patients with AD, it is important to look for the presence of agitation and a possible apparent cause. More specific antecedents to agitation include psychiatric disorders. In elderly patients, agitation may be exhibited in affective disorders, such as agitated depression, bipolar disorder, and involutional depression. Agitation also may be exhibited in various types of psychoses such as schizophrenia and paraphrenia, which has its onset in late life. In the early stages of the dementing illness, the patient can still make meaningful gestures or responses; however, in the advanced stages, the significance of agitation is much more inconspicuous, making an appropriate diagnosis more difficult. Overall, the precipitating and maintaining factors underlying agitation are numerous, but the psychiatric conditions discussed in this chapter (i.e., delirium, depression, psychosis, and anxiety) may be distinguished.

Delirium

Delirium is usually a transient, potentially catastrophic or life-threatening syndrome that indicates acute physiologic dysfunction of the cerebrum. *Dementia* is a chronically deteriorating process that signifies pathologic loss of neurons in the brain. Both of these disorders feature global cognitive impairment and thus overlap. Both can manifest as an agitated state. Agitation accompanied by confusion or psychosis often is caused by delirium. Agitated psychosis can also be secondary to the underlying dementia or caused by a chronic psychiatric condition such as schizophrenia or a mood disorder.

Delirium is often misdiagnosed as dementia, depression, or part of the normal aging process. This may be because of misconceptions about delirium, including the idea that it must be an agitated state; that emotional changes and irritability signify functional problems and thus rule out delirium; or that periods of lucidity mean the disorder is not organic (Lyness 1990). Although the term *sundowning* is typically used with patients with dementia to describe the phenomenon of agitation seemingly caused by darkness, it should not be considered synonymous with delirium, which is a psychiatric diagnosis and is not a description of behavior. Recent studies suggest that the sundowning phenomenon involves alterations of circadian rhythms and sensory inputs (Bliwise 1994). Delirious patients, in contrast to the common assumption of sundowning, are symptomatic during both day and night, although sensory deprivation at night certainly exacerbates delirium. Clarity is important because although sundowning is generally viewed as a benign problem, delirium actually results in considerable morbidity and mortality (Johnson et al. 1994). Signs and symptoms of delirium include changes in consciousness and cognition during a brief period. A reduced level of consciousness is manifested by an inability to focus, sustain, or shift attention. Cognitive abnormalities include disorientation, language difficulties, or impairments in learning and memory. Thinking is often fragmented and disjointed, as shown by rambling, irrelevant, or incoherent speech. These disturbances tend to fluctuate during the course of the day. Delirious patients may exhibit a wide array of psychiatric signs and symptoms, which include intermittent and labile symptoms of anxiety, irritability, agitation, aggression, fear, anger, depression, apathy, perplexity, suspiciousness, and euphoria. Perceptual disturbances such as illusions, delusions, and hallucinations commonly occur. They are usually fleeting, laden with emotion, and often bizarre. The sleep–wake cycle is invariably disrupted in patients with delirium; a patient may exhibit excessive drowsiness during the day and activity at night. These patients frequently become agitated when exposed to bright lights or noise. Sleep may be accompanied by nightmares, which may then merge into vivid hallucinations on awakening. The electrocardiogram (EEG) shows diffuse slow-wave or low-voltage activity in most delirious patients regardless of level of activity.

Clinically, there are three forms of delirium. In *hyperactive delirium*, which is typical of drug withdrawal, patients show increased psychomotor activity such as agitation, irritability, restlessness, rapid speech, and psychosis; may show disruptive behaviors such as screaming or resisting; and may sustain injuries from falling, combativeness, or pulling out intravascular lines. Patients with *hypoactive delirium*, which is typical of metabolic states, present with somnolence, apathy, slowed speech, and lethargy. This is the more common form but is easily overlooked and dismissed as a transient, insignificant problem. Strong stimuli are often needed for arousal, which is incomplete and transient at best. Patients with *mixed delirium* shift between hyperactive and hypoactive states.

A *catastrophic reaction* in a patient known to have dementia is essentially an agitated state brought on by environmental or psychological stress, often related to the relationship with the caregiver. Common precipitating factors are impatience, changing environments, blaming, and giving complicated orders. Although this type of reaction may resemble delirium, it is essentially different. The onset, duration, and attention features of delirium and catastrophic reaction are alike, but delirium usually lacks the environmental precipitant that characterizes catastrophic reactions, and a catastrophic reaction usually has no attendant EEG abnormalities (Tueth and Cheong 1993). The most reliable point of differentiation is response to psychosocial intervention. Providing reassurance, avoiding criticism, and reducing environmental stimuli and demands often help patients with dementia calm down relatively quickly. In a delirious patient, these psychosocial measures provide comfort but do not reverse the reaction (Tueth and Cheong 1993)

Common etiologic factors of delirium in elderly populations are electrolyte imbalances, dehydration, infections, hypoglycemia, hypoxia, and drug toxicity (e.g., anticholinergic drugs, sedative hypnotics, and narcotics). Susceptibility to these agents may depend on risk factors for delirium such as older age and compromised cognitive functioning, both of which are ordinarily present in the patient with dementia. Superimposed delirium is one of the principal diagnoses to consider when a patient with dementia suddenly exhibits an emergency behavioral complication (Lipowski 1989). Fluctuating manifestations between extreme confusion and periods of lucidity make delirium hard to detect, especially when clinicians spend only a short time with the patient, providing little opportunity to observe the cognitive changes during hospitalization. The differential diagnosis is critical because delirium is an acute medical emergency and dementia carries a quite different prognosis. In about 30%–50% of cases, delirium is superimposed on dementia, and both can cause agitation. These two conditions are differentiated by the sudden onset, brief duration, fluctuating course, inattention, and altered level of consciousness that are associated with delirium. Often the first feature of dementia is short-term memory defect in the absence of attentional deficit. Dementia is characterized by a slower onset, longer duration, stability over the course of the day, a steadily progressive course, and clear consciousness with intact attention until late stages. In dementia, lucid intervals are usually absent, perceptual disturbances are rare, and sleep is less disturbed. EEGs are normal in most cases of early dementia. Disorientation and memory impairment may be present with both conditions, and they may be absent in delirium. Thus, they are not useful in differential diagnosis. Moreover, not all rapid change in patients with dementia is caused by delirium. Other psychiatric illness, such as onset of paranoid delusions and catastrophic reactions to stressful situations, may cause these patients to deteriorate. However, because of the high prevalence of delirium in hospitalized elderly patients, any patient who may be manifesting agitation and shows decline in mental status is best presumed to be delirious until proven otherwise.

Because delirium often occurs in patients with serious medical illness, it contributes significantly to longer hospital stays, greater complications, and a high rate of short-term mortality. Hospital mortality has been reported to be from a 2- to 20-fold increase in patients with delirium compared with control groups of depressed, demented, or other medically ill patients (Francis 1990). Many authors assume that delirium is reversible when promptly diagnosed and treated, but reversibility is not part of the definition of delirium. Deteriorating physical function and cognition have been observed in long-term follow-up of patients experiencing delirium and possibly reflect progression of an unrecognized dementia that was "unmasked" by acute illness (Francis and Kapoor 1992). Maintaining a high index of suspicion may prevent many cases and arrest others at onset.

Depression

Depression coexisting with dementia is a clinical puzzle for clinicians who provide care to patients with dementia, especially those with AD. The wide variation in the prevalence of depression indicates the difficulty in the diagnosis of depression associated with dementia. In major depressive disorder, patients manifest a depressed mood, loss of interest or pleasure in all or most activities, significant change in appetite and body weight, insomnia or oversleeping, psychomotor agitation or retardation, inappropriate guilt or feelings of worthlessness, diminished concentration, and suicidal ideation. The neurovegetative signs and symptoms of depression may be a manifestation of the typical progression of AD; therefore, they cannot be relied on solely to make a diagnosis of a mood disorder. Clinicians must be aware of nonverbal cues of depression such as agitation, restlessness, passivity, verbal aggression, and vague somatic complaints. Unlike younger adults, depressed elderly people are more likely to manifest somatic complaints and hyperactive agitated behavior and delusions, and they are less likely to describe feelings of depression or express feelings of guilt. Depression is often masked when it is associated with preexisting neurological problems. Focal neurological abnormalities may be exacerbated by depression.

Determining the cause of agitation in the context of whether it is part of dementia or depression depends heavily on the psychiatrist's ability to elicit a thorough history, including information from collateral sources such as the patient's family and examination of the patient's mental state. One hurdle in examining depressive symptoms in elderly patients is how the clinician should regard the presence of vegetative symptoms in those who are medically ill and whether they should be considered symptoms of major depressive disorder. Clinicians can approach major depression as a syndrome that can be reliably recognized, allowing predictions about course, prognosis, and response to treatment. Demographic and biologic correlates of the syndrome can be delineated to postulate pathophysiological mechanisms and causes. For example, causes of the depressive syndrome may include primary affective disorder, grief, and vascular insults to the brain such as stroke. The other approach is to use the patient's life story. Learning the details of the patient's life and circumstances establishes the basis for supportive understanding of the person from which a healing relationship can develop (Jones and Reifleer 1994).

Although disturbed mood is the dominant characteristic of depression, patients may manifest cognitive deficits that mimic those of dementia. Various cognitive impairments that occur in patients with depression include impairments in learning, attention, memory, concentration, and visuospatial abilities. The combination of depression and cognitive impairments has sometimes been called the *dementia of depression,* implying that the cognitive symptoms are secondary to depression. Indications for such a secondary nature of the cognitive changes include a past history of affective disorder, an immediate history of depression preceding the appearance of dementia, a shorter duration of symptoms or significant fluctuations in the cognitive state from day to day or throughout the day, milder cognitive impairments, somatic delusions, negativism, and normal EEGs. Whether or not depression is present, the determination that significant cognitive decline has occurred warrants further medical investigation.

In some elderly patients, the cognitive impairment accompanying depression may be so severe that the patient may be thought to have a physical or organic brain syndrome. The most severe cases of depression tend to peak at 40–65 years of age, which is approximately the same time that dementias become clinically evident (Winstead et al. 1990). Patients with both dementia and depression may present with agitation, anxiety symptoms, or somatic complaints. To distinguish between depression and dementia in the presence of agitation, clinicians must consider the pattern of onset and the level of severity of the cognitive versus the affective symptoms. Persons with depression usually do not have long histories of memory loss, disorientation, incontinence, self-exposure, or loss of social tact. They are often irritable and hostile. They remain oriented at examination but often refuse to answer questions and may become angry. Their family is usually aware of the illness. The onset of depression is dated and more acute, symptoms are of short duration with rapid progression, and patients have a family history of affective disorder. There is an identifiable onset of cognitive impairment, both in terms of time and emotionally important life events, such as loss of employment or loss of a spouse. Patients with depression usually complain of their cognitive deficits in detail, feel distressed, and seek help. They highlight their failures, make little effort to do tasks, and do not try to keep up. In elderly patients with depression, affective symptoms are pervasive, and their behavior is incongruent with cognitive dysfunction. On examination, these patients usually do not exhibit sundowning behavior. "I don't know" answers are typical, recent and remote memory loss are similar, decreased memory for specific periods is common, attention and concentration are preserved, and primitive reflexes are absent.

In contrast, patients with dementia cannot relate appropriately to their physicians during evaluation. They attempt to answer questions with irrelevant, nonsensical, or confabulatory answers. They do not complain of their cognitive deficits but rather conceal them, and their complaints are nonspecific and appear unconcerned. The patient usually delights in his or her accomplishments, struggles with tasks, relies on notes and calendars, and has no family history of depression. The patient's affect is labile and shallow and his or her behavior is usually compatible with cognitive impairment. Examination shows evidence of primitive reflexes, perseveration, or other neurological deficits. Cognitive impairment is broad based and includes problems in orientation, recent memory, intellectual functioning, and ability to abstract (Yesavage 1992). The patient with dementia has no gaps in memory, has faulty attention and concentration, gives frequent "near-miss" answers, and shows sundowning behavior. The patient's family is usually unaware of the slowly progressing dementing illness. The onset is broadly and vaguely dated with a family history of AD.

It is imperative to evaluate the course and manifestations of other psychopathologic symptoms in patients with both depression and dementia because such patients may frequently have other psychiatric symptoms and syndromes and may take various psychotropic agents that may further complicate the clinical picture (Alexopoulos and Abrams 1991). Clinicians should always judge whether the depression is a primary clinical problem. For example, a patient with dementia in whom hypersomnia, anhedonia, and even depressed mood develops after he or she is treated with benzodiazepines for agitated behavior may be suffering from the side effects of these drugs and may not be suitable for antidepressant treatment. On the other hand, depression may lead to behavioral symptoms such as agitation or a tendency to resist care. Clinicians may erroneously treat the agitation with antipsychotic agents without paying attention to the underlying depression. In some elderly patients with depression, anxiety may be the most prominent symptom. Although attribution of anxiety symptoms to depression should be strongly considered, medical causes for symptoms must be investigated.

When depression coexists with dementia, the important step is to determine whether its magnitude or severity warrant therapeutic intervention. Accurately diagnosing major depression is most crucial because of its responsiveness to treatment and its association with morbidity and mortality when untreated. Although reversible dementia can be suspected in depressed patients with marked agitation, in most cases the distinction can only be made after antidepressant treatment has been instituted.

Psychosis

Patients with psychosis have a gross impairment in reality testing, frequently manifested by hallucinations and delusions. Although psychosis is seen often in patients with a major mental illness, such as schizophrenia or bipolar disorder, there are several other causes of psychosis. For example, psychosis and behavioral disturbances frequently manifest as comorbidities of AD. Dementia can present with various psychiatric symptoms such as delusions, hallucinations, depression, agitation, aggression, and apathy. These are important determinants of patient morbidity that frequently cause significant burden to caregivers and may lead to institutionalization. In a nursing home sample, delusions and hallucinations resulted in more frequent and severe behavioral disorders such as agitation and combativeness (Rovner et al. 1986).

Behavioral disturbances can be a reaction to the subjective experience of a hallucination or delusion, which may be difficult to evaluate directly. It is also difficult to separate formal thought disorder from aphasia because some degree of aphasia invariably develops with progression of the disease. Psychotic features may be associated with a rapidly progressive course of illness (Jeste et al. 1992). In evaluating psychotic symptoms in patients with AD, it is important to determine whether bizarre behavior or speech may be secondary to other factors such as confusion or cognitive impairment (Lopez et al. 1991). A person with minimal insight who has a memory problem may, for example, misinterpret his forgetfulness and believe that someone is moving or stealing his belongings.

Delusions are false, strongly held personal beliefs based on incorrect inferences about reality from which a patient cannot be dissuaded. Delusional beliefs may be categorized as persecutory, misidentification syndromes, and of other types. Strongly held beliefs not amounting to delusional strength (overvalued ideas) also appear in those who have AD. The most commonly described psychotic symptoms in AD are persecutory delusions. The frequency of persecutory delusions in patients with AD varies from 10%–73%. Specifically, themes of theft, suspiciousness, and threats of bodily harm are most commonly reported. Such patients usually make accusations that their money or belongings have been stolen. They may be focused on the idea that someone is trying to harm them or plot against them. Occasionally, these patients may develop more systematized delusions, as in erotomania. Experts say that poor memory is often the core cause of these paranoid ideas; delusional explanations replace memory for misplaced articles and the forgotten identity of individuals. These false beliefs are different in content, form, and intensity from delusions that are characteristic of patients with schizophrenia. Delusions of thought control and somatic, nihilistic, and grandiose delusions are rarely reported in patients with both schizophrenia and major depressive disorder (Deutsch et al. 1991). Delusions in those with dementia are inversely related to cortical atrophy (Jacoby and Levy 1980), which indicates that intact cortical functions are a requisite for delusions to be experienced.

Misidentification syndromes occur in approximately 25% of patients with AD (Rabin et al. 1988). Misidentifications are false beliefs that appear to be secondary to gnostic deficits such that patients do not recognize their homes, caregivers, or themselves. The most common types of misidentifications are the belief that other people are living in the patient's home; the belief that people seen on television are real and are in the room; and the misidentification of the patient's own reflection in the mirror. These false beliefs can be the cause of the aggressive disturbances in the patient with dementia and are often the reason for the demoralization of the caregiver.

Hallucinations are not as common as other psychotic symptoms in patients with AD, with the reported frequency ranging from 21%–49% of those evaluated. Prevalence rates vary with the population sampled, the basis for making the AD diagnosis, and the severity of the illness. Visual hallucinations tend to occur more frequently than auditory ones (Wragg and Jeste 1989). During the evaluation of these patients, it is important to look for signs of sensory deprivation, such as deafness or cataract, which may contribute to perceptual problems. Hallucinations are frequently fragmented and disorganized. Whereas visual hallucinations usually involve seeing imaginary people or animals, auditory hallucinations are often accompanied by conversations with the imagined voices. Sometimes the two types overlap, particularly when the vision is seen through a window or in a room that is not brightly lit (Tueth 1995). Redirection and reassurance are sometimes ineffective when agitation results from hallucinations, thus making caregivers feel helpless.

Psychotic symptoms have been described in association with the presence of bradykinesia, rigidity, tremor, postural and gait changes, and changes in facial expression (Mayeux et al. 1985). When subjects with dementia of the Alzheimer type were divided by the presence or absence of extrapyramidal signs (EPS), the groups with EPS were more likely to have delusions and hallucinations.

It is important to determine whether psychosis is part of the dementia or a primary psychotic disorder. Studies indicate that up to 12% of nursing home residents suffer from schizophrenia or other primary psychotic disorders. The presence of psychotic symptoms in elderly patients, especially in nursing homes, poses a diagnostic challenge. DSM-IV-TR (American Psychiatric Association 2000) criteria for schizophrenia require the presence of at least two characteristic symptoms during a 1-month period, such as hallucinations, delusions, disorganized speech or behavior, and negative symptoms; significant social or occupational dysfunction after onset of the illness; continuous signs of the illness for at least 6 months; and exclusion of substances or general medical conditions as possible causative agents. Older patients with schizophrenia may present with long histories of the illness because it typically begins during young adulthood. However, many elderly persons present with new onset of psychotic symptoms in late life. There are several medical and neurological disorders that can present with psychotic symptoms in late life. Because schizophrenia lacks pathognomonic signs or characteristic radiographic and laboratory findings, it is important to rule out other possible causes of psychosis.

Considerable overlap exists between late-onset schizophrenia and delusional disorder, which also has its onset in middle to late adult life. However, DSM-IV-TR (American Psychiatric Association 2000) criteria for delusional disorder specify the presence of nonbizarre delusions, tactile or olfactory hallucinations related to the delusional theme, and no marked impairment in psychosocial functioning.

Anxiety

Anxiety is defined as worry, apprehension, or panic that occurs in the absence of—or is out of proportion to—an actual threat. Such reactions are often accompanied by unpleasant autonomic nervous system arousal. Symptoms of sympathetic arousal include tachycardia, tremor, hyperventilation, lightheadedness, inner tremulousness, and unsteadiness. Less common are complaints of "nerves" or fearfulness. Whereas fear is more engendered by an external threat, such as being physically attacked, anxiety is an emotional response that is inappropriate to the reality of the external stimulus. True anxiety or panic episodes often precipitate visits to the emergency room, where electrocardiography, blood gas studies, and (at times) neuroimaging studies are done to rule out acute cardiovascular or neurological disease.

Estimates of the prevalence of anxiety among elderly patients may be spuriously low because of lack of recognition or misdiagnosis as biological illness. However, the number of anxiety-related complaints heard by primary physicians from elderly patients may actually be higher. Anxious, agitated, or delirious patients are often either ignored or labeled as "difficult." The commonly diagnosed anxiety disorders such as panic disorder, posttraumatic stress disorder, generalized anxiety disorder, phobic illness, and obsessive-compulsive disorder may be only the tip of the symptomatic iceberg. When ignored, anxiety and fear in an increasingly emotionally exhausted patient can tip the physiological scale in a negative direction.

Anxiety can produce disturbances in cognitive functions of perceiving, thinking, and conceptualizing. An anxious elderly person may be easily distracted, may appear confused, may have difficulty remembering events, may experience inability to think clearly, and may lose his or her objectivity, thus making it hard to tease out anxiety disorders from agitation caused by dementia, especially if the symptoms are accompanied by other behavioral disturbances. Anxious patients may attempt to control their surroundings, may resist care, or may make unrealistic demands for attention. To appropriately differentiate an anxiety disorder from agitation in dementia, the clinician should perform a thorough evaluation that includes a description of the current symptoms, previous episodes, other psychiatric history, medical conditions, current and previous medications, life or situational changes, and history of alcohol use. A physical examination should focus on the stigmas of the physical causes of anxiety, and laboratory screening should be done to investigate suspected medical conditions.

Aside from the psychiatric conditions that may be associated with anxiety—dementia, depressive disorders, mania, adjustment disorder with anxious mood, schizophrenia and related disorders, somatoform disorders, and personality disorders—several medical conditions are increasingly associated with complaints of anxiety in elderly patients. Some of the more common medical conditions associated with anxiety include hyperthyroidism, pheochromocytoma, diabetes mellitus, mitral valve prolapse, chronic obstructive lung disease, temporal lobe epilepsy, Parkinson's disease, and carcinoid syndrome. Pharmacological agents commonly associated with precipitation of anxiety include sympathomimetics, methylxanthines, steroids, thyroid hormone, and anticholinergics. Withdrawal from alcohol, caffeine, benzodiazepines, and tobacco is also anxiogenic. Additional investigation should be made into areas of situational stress, loss, or conflict. When the number or intensity of stressors increases, dysfunctional behaviors such as agitation occur. Adaptational stressors may include an experience of displacement or sudden loss such as a move to a nursing home or the death of a spouse, retirement, or a major change in physical health. Stressors related to the environment may cause considerable anxiety associated with negative life events such as the lack of social support, economic problems, and difficulties with mobility or transportation (Martin et al. 1995).

Conclusions

Patients with AD exhibit various neuropsychiatric disturbances. Agitation is common and may be regarded as a common behavioral pathway for a patient with dementia who seems to have a restricted response to a wide array of internal and external stimuli. Elderly patients with cognitive deficits along with the attendant behavioral disturbances of dementia pose significant diagnostic and treatment challenges to clinicians. To meet these challenges, clinicians must maintain a systematic and thoughtful approach each time, taking advantage of available technology as well as exercising full insight.

Case Example

A 68-year-old woman was brought to the emergency department because of shortness of breath and increasing agitation since the death of her husband 2 days earlier. She was subsequently admitted to the hospital for pneumonia. She had a long history of chronic obstructive pulmonary disease. The previous night, she had panicked, pointed at the curtain, and screamed that someone was coming in the window. While in the hospital, the patient misidentified one of the nurse's aides as her dead husband, and she defecated in the bed. When her son tried to comfort her, she did not recognize him. After consultation, sedating medications were given. The patient's condition worsened, with persistent daytime somnolence and nighttime agitation. Her primary care physician began to suspect delirium. Aggressive pulmonary treatments were initiated, and discontinuation of the sedating medications corrected her hypoxemia. As her medical condition stabilized, the delirium cleared completely.

The physician should ask family members and nursing staff about the patient's baseline level of function and any recent mental changes. The present history is also important for identifying any acute medical condition. Knowing the patient's medical history, use of medications, and social habits helps clinicians differentiate causes of agitation and, in this case, identify possible causes of delirium.

References

Alexopoulos GS, Abrams RC: Depression in Alzheimer's disease. Psychiatr Clin North Am 14:327–339, 1991

American Psychiatric Association: Diagnostic and Statistical Manual of Mental Disorders, 4th Edition Text Revision. Washington, DC, American Psychiatric Association, 2000

Bliwise DI: What is sundowning? J Am Geriatr Soc 42:1009–1011, 1994

Deutsch LH, Bylsma FW, Rovner BW, et al: Psychosis and physical aggression in probable Alzheimer's disease. Am J Psychiatry 148:1159–1163, 1991

Francis J, Kapoor WN: Delirium in hospitalized elderly. J Gen Intern Med 5:65–79, 1990

Francis J, Kapoor WN: Prognosis after hospital discharge of older medical patients with delirium. J Am Geriatr Soc 0:601–606, 1992

Jacoby R, Levy R: Computed tomography in the elderly, 2: senile dementia: diagnosis and functional impairment. Br J Psychiatry 136:256–269, 1980

Jeste DS, Wragg RE, Salmon DP, et al: Cognitive deficits of patients with Alzheimer's disease with and without delusions. Am J Psychiatry 149:184–189, 1992

Johnson J, Sims R, Gottlieb G: Differential diagnosis of dementia, delirium and depression. Drugs and Aging 5:431–444, 1994

Jones BN, Reifleer BV: Depression coexisting with dementia. Med Clin North Am 78:823–839, 1994

Lipowski ZJ: Delirium in the elderly patients. N Engl J Med 320:578–582, 1989

Lopez OL, Becker JT, Brenner RP, et al: Alzheimer's disease with delusions and hallucinations: neuropsychological and electroencephalographic correlates. Neurology 41:906–912, 1991

Lyness JM: Delirium: Masquerades and misdiagnosis in elderly inpatients. J Am Geriatr Soc 38:1235–1238, 1990

Martin LM, Fleming KC, Evans JM: Recognition and management of anxiety and depression in elderly patients. Mayo Clin Proc 70:999–1006, 1995

Mayeux R, Stern Y, Spanton S: Heterogeneity in dementia of the Alzheimer type: evidence for subgroups. Neurology 35:453–461, 1985

Rabin EH, Drevets WC, Burke WJ: The nature of psychotic symptoms in senile dementia of the Alzheimer type. J Geriatr Psychiatry Neurol 1:16–20, 1988

Roper JM, Shapira J, Chang BL, et al: Agitation in the demented patient: a framework for management. J Gerontol Nurs 17:17–21, 1991

Rovner BW, Kafonek S, Filipp L, et al: Prevalence of mental illness in a community nursing home. Am J Psychiatry 143:11, 1986

Tueth MJ: How to manage depression and psychosis in Alzheimer's disease. Geriatrics 50:43–49, 1995

Tueth MJ, Cheong JA: Delirium: diagnosis and treatment in the older patient. Geriatrics 48:75–80, 1993

Winstead DK, Mielke DH, O'Neill PT: Diagnosis and treatment of depression in the elderly: a review. Psychiatr Med 8:85–98, 1990

Wragg RE, Jeste DV: Overview of depression and psychosis in Alzheimer's disease. Am J Psychiatry 146:577–587, 1989

Yesavage JA: Depression in the elderly. Postgrad Med 91:255–261, 1992

CHAPTER 6

Clinical Assessment and Management of Agitation in Residential Settings

Susan Eller, M.A., R.N.
Linda Griffin, R.N.C.
Christine Mote, M.S.N., R.N.C.S.

P atients who are easily agitated and who are at high risk for becoming physically aggressive can become a threat to any unit and hinder the well-being of all. It is important to establish a safe environment in which to care for these individuals. With good assessment skills and a positive approach, nursing home teams are able to develop a successful treatment plan to manage patients with aggressive and combative behavior.

Recognition of Aggression

General Guidelines

The short-term goal should be to reduce and eventually eliminate inappropriate aggression. A well-trained staff is able to achieve this goal by being able to recognize early signs of agitation, possible causes of aggressive behavior, characteristics of aggressive or combative residents, the need for a comprehensive multidisciplinary assessment, and appropriate intervention and goals.

Manifestation of Aggression

Agitation in patients with dementia can manifest in various ways:

- An old and frightened woman is unable to sit still for more than 30 seconds. She runs for the door, yelling in a high, shrill voice, "Help me, help me. I'm so scared." She is a difficult patient to manage and is eliciting numerous complaints from other patients and their families.
- An elderly gentleman sits in a chair. He is slapping his face repeatedly. He has also become physically aggressive with the nursing home staff and other patients. The staff members believe they can no longer care for him.
- A healthy 62-year-old man diagnosed with Alzheimer's disease 2 years earlier tries to go home every night, promising to return in the morning. When the nursing home staff does not allow this, he becomes agitated and upset, which leads to physical altercations. He also has difficulty understanding why other patients become upset when he tries to turn their chairs over to work on them. He used to be a carpenter, so he wonders why it is a problem for him to work.
- A disheveled elderly woman roams in and out of other residents' rooms, gathering belongings as she goes. She becomes tearful and upset when the staff takes away the belongings and returns them to their rightful owners. Other patients and their families complain about this behavior. The woman is in danger of being evicted from the nursing home because of her behavior.

Variations in Behavior

Screaming, wandering, rummaging, and becoming physically aggressive are all characteristics of patients with agitation (Robinson et al. 1968). However, not all patients display all of these behaviors, and there can be differences in the intensity of the behavior. For example, either frustration at being unable to perform activities that were once commonplace or confusion about their surroundings can cause patients with dementia to become agitated. Some patients experience a constant state of anxiety, and others become anxious to the point of agitation when they are overwhelmed or overstimulated by something in the environment (Robinson et al. 1968). Most of the agitation and irritability reactions are very spontaneous and short lived. Such episodes are most often reflex actions to frustrating situations (Crisis Prevention Institute 1987).

These episodes should not be taken personally by the staff. They often occur in the course of confusion and misinterpretation. An example of a typical episode is that of a patient walking down the hall, half dressed, going to breakfast. He is stopped by a staff member who attempts to redirect him back to his room to finish dressing. The patient does not understand this intervention and does not realize his attire is inappropriate for the situation. He physically resists, striking out at the staff member and cursing.

In many cases, the subsequent escalation or defusing of the patient's behavior may depend entirely on how the staff reacts (Crisis Prevention Institute 1987). If the staff member allows him- or herself to become irrational or unprofessional, he or she will ultimately find his attempts at de-escalation frustrated.

Contributing Etiologic Factors

Environmental Considerations

The environment is the first aspect to consider when determining the contributing causes of agitation in a nursing home. Sometimes eliminating environmental stimulation reduces or eliminates agitation, but this basic solution is often overlooked. Important environmental factors to consider include the following:

> **Unfamiliar people, places, or sounds.** Moving into a nursing home can be very traumatic to a patient. Being unable to recognize surroundings can provoke anxiety. Often the nursing home is very noisy, with many unfamiliar sounds, including overhead paging, piped-in music, and other patients calling out. These stimuli can also provoke anxiety in patients. The differences are enormous between living in a private home and living in an extended-care facility. In contrast to a private setting, nursing home patients are forced to come into contact with a large number of people, including nursing staff, housekeepers, dieticians, maintenance workers, physicians, families, and other residents. This can be overwhelming for patients and can be a major factor in the development of agitation (Calkins et al. 1988).
>
> **Sensory overload.** Sensory overload is also a primary cause of agitation in nursing home patients. The noise and activity levels mentioned previously can also be overstimulating to patients. Patients often have very little opportunity for solitude and privacy. This can add to the stress level of the patient and cause agitation (Calkins et al. 1988).
>
> **Changes in routine.** Entering a nursing home is a complete change in lifestyle for most patients and can be very a difficult adjustment. Basic routines, such as meal times, bathing, and bedtime, are now dictated by

the institution's standards. Imagine the frustration of a patient who has gone to bed at 11:00 P.M. for the past 25 years but must now go to bed at 9:00 P.M. Consider the indignity of being bathed by an unfamiliar staff member, who is often very rushed because of his or her heavy workload. Additionally, food choices are often limited, although good nutrition is a priority for most institutions.

Isolation. Although overstimulation may become problematic, there is also a considerable amount of isolation in nursing homes. Patients often feel lost and abandoned, causing them to feel severe anxiety and even act out on feelings of anger. Because of cognitive deficits, many patients are unsure as to why they are living in a new environment. Familiar faces are absent, and patients may have nothing in common with their peers. Staff continuity is often a problem, resulting in patients' not being cared for by the same person from day to day.

Physiological and Psychological Considerations

Because of their age, nursing home patients are especially vulnerable to many physical complications. It is essential that each patient receive a comprehensive physical and neurological examination on admission (Gruetzner 1988).

Simple problems such as sleep deprivation or disturbed sleep patterns may lead to fatigue and irritability that, if left untreated, can escalate into uncontrolled behavior. A more serious sleep problem occurs when a patient is sleeping during the day and is awake all night. This can cause the patient to become confused and difficult to redirect and may ultimately lead to problematic behavior. Physical discomfort is another area often overlooked because of patients' inabilities to communicate thoughts and feelings. Pain, fever, constipation, urinary retention, and fecal impaction are just a few of the physical manifestations that can precipitate behavior problems. Visual or auditory impairment can also have an impact on a patient's ability to cope with his or her environment.

Psychiatric manifestations of mental illness, such as visual or auditory hallucinations, delusional thoughts, paranoia, and other thought disorders, can lead to the misinterpretation by patients of their surroundings and to inappropriate behavior (Gruetzner 1988). Adverse side effects from medication can produce signs that may be perceived as agitation by a caregiver or even the patient (Gruetzner 1988). For example, increased pacing, restlessness, rocking movements, irritability, or a report of feeling "jumpy on the inside" may be the result of akathesia rather than signs of agitation. Many clinicians mistake this side effect for agitation and increase the amount of medication the resident is taking. This can result in a worsening in the behavior or lead to additional adverse side effects.

Delirium is an acute brain syndrome associated with excitement and agitation. It is nearly always associated with drug intoxication or medical, surgical, or neurological disorders (Gruetzner 1988). Delirium should be diagnosed through physical examination and tests. The condition may be resolved when treated promptly and correctly. However, if left untreated, it may result in death.

Functional Considerations

Agitation can also be caused by interactions between the patient and other individuals, such as staff, family members, or other patients. Patients with dementing illnesses often have difficulty communicating with others. They become frustrated when asked too many questions, given directions too quickly, asked to do tasks that are too complex, or hurried through tasks. It is difficult for these patients to make decisions. Choosing clothing for the day or deciding what to eat can be overwhelming. This can lead to acting-out behavior that can persist throughout the day. Loud voices, high stress, or abrupt movements can be perceived as threatening, leading to altercations. These patients usually respond poorly to critical remarks, condescending manners, and other types of confrontational behavior. Sudden unexpected physical contact can also elicit a fight-or-flight response in (Robinson et al. 1968).

Prevention Strategies

Assessment

The key to managing agitation is prevention. Preventive management means ongoing assessment and anticipatory actions (Crisis Prevention Institute 1987). Patients should be assessed on a regular basis. Agitated behaviors should be noted and discussed in an effort to identify the cause of the behavior. Assessing the situation is the most important intervention in the deescalation process. Assessment involves a rapid evaluation of the facts at hand. The following question needs to be asked: "What behaviors are being demonstrated?" Intense anxiety, verbal assault, and physical aggression must be recognized for the intervention to be effective (Crisis Prevention Institute 1987).

Identifying these changes in the early stages and with the appropriate staff intervention can eliminate crisis situations (Crisis Prevention Institute 1987). Assessment of anxiety is important because it is often the first observable level of agitation. This may present as a disheveled appearance, restlessness, handwringing, facial grimacing, repetitive movements, rapid speech, confusion, or even the appearance of being in pain (Robinson et al. 1968). Staff response should be to assess and acknowledge these changes.

Spending time with the patient and offering either assistance or support can stop the situation from escalating. Assessment of anxiety in the agitated patient with dementia is best conceptualized as a change in behavior. The use of the ABC mnemonic can help with identifying the components of anxiety: Is there a change in *appearance* (A)?; Is there a change in *behavior* (B)?; and Is there a change in *comfort level* (C)? In some instances, the patient's anxiety may not have been recognized or was missed by the staff. The patient may now become verbally aggressive and may begin shouting and cursing, act in an accusatory fashion, and may become verbally threatening. If safety is not an issue, the best intervention is to allow the patient to verbalize his or her thoughts. Staff members should not argue, become defensive, or threaten the patient. Asking the patient to calm down so the situation can be discussed is an appropriate intervention. Directions should always be given in a calm, clear manner. At times, the situation may escalate into a crisis in which a patient may become physically aggressive. Staff members must be trained to respond correctly to such crises to protect patients and themselves.

Team Approach

A multidisciplinary approach is essential for the prevention of agitation. The team should consist of the primary caregivers, social worker, physician (or physicians), and family members. The patient should also be involved whenever possible. The entire team should participate in a thorough assessment that must include physical, neurological, and psychosocial examinations. These elements are necessary for the development of a treatment plan that is both comprehensive and achievable.

Psychosocial Aspects

Although the physical assessment is very important, understanding the psychosocial aspects of a patient's life is just as important. Lifestyle, home environment, career, relationships, financial resources, recreational preferences, and coping skills are vital in the development of the treatment plan. The treatment team's goal is to become familiar with the individual's moods, strengths, and weaknesses and how he or she reacts to change. It is important to remember to treat this person in a holistic manner; the patient should be treated as a whole person and not just as a behavioral problem.

Rapport

Prevention can also be maintained by developing a good rapport with the patient. This needs to begin on the day the patient is admitted to the facility. Empathy is the key here, with staff members being aware of the enormous changes occurring in this individual's life and his or her uncertainty of the future. Taking the time to establish rapport can prevent a catastrophic reaction later. Developing a relationship with the patient can also help in reducing feelings of isolation and give reassurance that someone cares and is looking out for the patient's well being.

Flexibility

Flexibility is another important factor when treating cognitively impaired patients. Although structure is necessary in providing good care, there are also occasions when the patient's emotional status must be taken into consideration. At these times, it can be beneficial to alter schedules. For example, some patients have been accustomed to sleeping until 9 A.M. for the past 30 years. They can become very upset when awakened at 6 A.M. and cannot understand the need for the rigid schedule. Another example is that of a wandering patient who refuses to sit in the dining room for meals; this individual is able to get an adequate nutritional intake when the staff provides finger foods for him and allows him to graze for several hours.

Allowing for individual idiosyncrasies can mean the difference between a calm and an agitated patient. Helping the patient to feel successful in his or her environment is also a goal for the prevention of agitation. These patients often have difficulty coping with the challenges they face. As their cognitive abilities decline, their emotional responses are magnified.

Self-Esteem

Self-esteem in elderly patients with dementia is an ongoing issue. An inability to perform tasks that were previously simple contributes to insecurity and frustration. It is important to provide cognitively impaired patients with tasks that enhance their sense of personal integrity while not overtaxing their mental capabilities (Hellen 1992). An example of this is to offer choices but to limit the number of choices; this helps to keep the decision-making process manageable. Minimizing the differences between the choices is also helpful. For example, it is better to make a statement such as: "You may have an apple or an orange." Asking a question such as: "Would you like an apple or an orange?" can cause confusion by requiring the patient to make a choice between different items. In this case, the patient must first decide if he or she wants fruit or not by answering "yes or no." Secondly, the patient must decide which fruit he or she wants, an apple or an orange.

Meaningful Activities

Another means of preventing agitation is involving the individual in meaningful activities that relate, however remotely, to past responsibilities (Hellen 1992). Allowing a former homemaker to assist with folding the laundry or a former foreman to carry a clipboard to monitor the "progress of the floor" can be invaluable in helping the patient maintain his or her self-esteem and self-worth. Simplifying tasks by breaking them into manageable increments allows the patient to continue his or her daily activities despite declining functional abilities (Hellen 1992). Tailoring activities and tasks to suit the patient's abilities can help that person better use his or her strengths to overcome deficits.

Environment

Managing the environment correctly can lead to calmer patients and happier staff members. The team should strive for a 60%–80% success rate in tasks given to patients with dementing illnesses (Hellen 1992).

Communication

Good communications skills can also serve to prevent agitation. Key points to remember are as follows:

• Approach the patient in a warm, friendly manner.
• Speak slowly and clearly.
• Use short, simple sentences.
• Approach the patient face forward, so as not to startle.
• Use the patient's name to maintain rapport.
• Do not argue or go into lengthy explanations.
• Watch for nonverbal cues of increasing anxiety.
• If patient appears anxious, back off and reapproach when calm.
• Use cues such as signs, pictures, or photographs.
• To enhance communication, be sensitive to the patient's mood, facial expression, and body language.

Additional Considerations

Considerations that can prevent, reduce, or manage agitation include the following:

- Providing a safe area for patients to pace or wander to relieve built-up tension
- Keeping the environment, such as the patient's room, free of clutter and keeping the furniture arranged in a consistent fashion
- Keeping a log of the patient's outbursts to assist in identifying patterns and triggers
- Using good communication between staff members about pertinent information that can be used to prevent incidents of agitation in specific patients
- Planning tasks and activities around the best time of the day for each individual (e.g., some people are morning people and others are night people)
- Recognizing patients' boredom and allowing them to assist with simple tasks (e.g., making rounds with staff, delivering mail, transporting residents)
- Educating staff members on the importance of using distraction (e.g., looking at magazines, books, talking with peers, walking) as a therapeutic tool
- In extended-care facilities, having a quiet room or area where agitated patients can be alone to regain control and avoid catastrophic reactions
- Using diversional activities, such as pet therapy, music therapy, art therapy, or gardening, which are beneficial and therapeutic
- Educating the staff on the developmental stages of older adults to enhance the quality care for the patients

Physical Interventions

Physical interventions should be used as a last resort. These interventions are used to control a patient until he or she can regain control of him- or herself. Interventions in this area must be done in accordance with the facility's policy (Crisis Prevention Institute 1987). Each situation must be evaluated on an individual basis, looking at the facts in an objective manner. Was the cause of the agitation something that could have been prevented? Did the environment need to be changed? Did the patient's routine need to be altered? Would a change in approach have made a difference?

After exhausting all nonmedical interventions, medication may required. This should be used cautiously and with close medical supervision. After the incident has occurred, a debriefing session with all staff involved, including the patient if appropriate, should take place. It is important for both the staff members and the patient that closure takes place so that episodes and crises can be resolved and so that the interventions will not be seen as punitive.

Conclusions

Many agitated patients with dementia can be very hard to manage. This can lead to frustration and burnout on the part of the staff and caregivers. These patients are not always responsible for their behaviors. It is vital that educational opportunities and support are provided for caregivers. In order for them to give quality care, staff members must feel competent with their abilities to perform their duties in a professional manner. It is up to us as educators and caregivers to give these patients the care and respect they deserve.

References

Calkins, MP, Arch M: Design for Dementia: Planning Environments for the Elderly and Confused. Owings Mills, MD, National Health Publishing, 1988, pp 118–126

Crisis Prevention Institute: Nonviolent Crisis Intervention. Brookfield, WI, Crisis Prevention Institute, 1987

Gruetzner H: Alzheimer's: A Caregiver's Guide and Sourcebook. New York, Wiley & Sons, 1988

Hellen CR: Alzheimer's Disease: Activity-Focused Care. Stoneham, MA, Butterworth-Heinemann, 1992, pp 71–75

Robinson A, Spencer B, White L: Understanding Difficult Behaviors: Some Practical Suggestions for Coping with Alzheimer's Disease and Related Illnesses. Ypsilanti, MI, Eastern Michigan University, 1968

Nursing Care Adaptations, Behavioral Interventions, Environmental Changes, and Sensory Enhancement

Conceptual, Process, and Outcome Issues

Perla Werner, Ph.D.

For many years, psychoactive medications and physical restraints have constituted the primary approach in the management of patients with agitation (Cohen-Mansfield et al. 1993; Fleming and Evans 1995; Sky and Grossberg 1994; Weinrich et al. 1995). Within the past decade, however, nonpharmacological interventions have been recognized as viable ways to treat agitation. The development and implementation of this type of treatment have been identified by medical and nursing staff members, researchers, and legislators as important matters. The Omnibus Reconciliation Act of 1987 (OBRA '87) mandates not only a reduction in the use of chemical and physical restraints but also the development of nursing interventions for the management of behavioral problems in cognitively impaired nursing home residents. The National Institute on Aging, recognizing the need to advance a research agenda for the development of behavioral approaches to the treatment of agitation in dementia, organized a special workshop aimed at identifying "the most important scientific problems and questions in the development of behavioral approaches to treatment and management" (Radebaugh et al. 1996, p. 8).

The purpose of this chapter is to synthesize the status of research on nonpharmacological interventions for the management of agitation in elderly persons with dementia. It is not intended to be an exhaustive review of this area; rather, it is meant to discuss and focus on the main conceptual, process, and outcome issues involved in the development and implementation of these interventions.

Conceptual Issues

Before examining specific interventions and reviewing their usefulness and efficacy, it is necessary to identify the conceptual framework that guides their implementation. Conceptual issues include the definition of the concept under study as well as the theoretical approach used.

Definition of the Concept

Although varied systems exist for classifying agitated behaviors, there is ample consensus today that agitation includes several syndromes. Cohen-Mansfield and Billig (1986) have provided the first and most widely recognized operational definition of agitation. According to this definition, *agitation* includes inappropriate verbal, vocal, or motor activity that is not explained by needs or confusion.

Empirically, three agitation factors or syndromes have been identified: 1) aggressive behaviors such as hitting, kicking, pushing, grabbing, and tearing; 2) physically nonaggressive behaviors such as pacing inappropriately, robing and disrobing, handling things inappropriately, repetitious mannerisms, and general restlessness; and 3) verbally agitated behaviors such as constant requests for attention, negativism, and screaming (Cohen-Mansfield et al. 1994). Each syndrome is associated with different etiologies (for a review of the correlates of agitated behaviors, see Cohen-Mansfield et al. 1994) and, therefore, with different interventions (Cohen-Mansfield and Werner 1994).

Theoretical Approach Used for the Development of Interventions

The theoretical basis influences the management mode (pharmacological or nonpharmacological) as well as the content (e.g., behavior management, environmental change, caregiver training and education) of interventions. Various explanations for the occurrence of agitation have been proposed:

1. **Agitation associated with neurological factors.** According to this approach, agitation results from the primary degenerative processes

occurring in the brain as a consequence of the dementia (Franzen and Martin 1996; Jeste and Krull 1991). Numerous researchers have indeed found clear relationships between agitated behaviors and cognitive impairment (for a review, see Cohen-Mansfield et al. 1996).

Lately, a growing body of research has linked agitated behaviors to the involvement of neurotransmitters. Dementia, and particularly Alzheimer's disease, is associated with the loss of cholinergic neurons and neurotransmitters, including 5-HT (Kumar et al. 1995). Dysfunction in the serotonergic system has been associated with the appearance of agitated behavior in general and physically aggressive behavior in particular (Mintzer and Brawman-Mintzer 1996).

The neurological deterioration that accompanies the dementing process may cause disinhibition in the form of verbally or physically aggressive agitation (Cohen-Mansfield and Werner 1997). Alternatively, agitation may be understood as an attempt to communicate and express feelings given the gradual loss of language and social skills associated with the dementing process (Carlson et al. 1995).

2. **Agitation associated with medical factors.** Similar to other elderly persons, those with dementia present multiple chronic conditions, including arthritis, hypertension, gastrointestinal and genitourinary diseases, and psychiatric disorders (e.g., anxiety disorder, paranoia or delusional disorder) (Segal 1996). These conditions may function as precipitants of agitation either directly or through the pain, psychiatric discomfort, and distress associated with them.

   In a study aimed at examining the effectiveness of three nonpharmacological interventions for the management of verbally disruptive behaviors in nursing home residents (Cohen-Mansfield and Werner 1997), one-quarter of the verbally agitated residents who underwent a thorough medical examination displayed physiological signs of pain. It is important, therefore, to rule out an organic etiology before initiating a treatment for agitation (see "Process Issues" discussion later in the chapter).

   Basic to this theoretical explanation is the presumption that agitation, which is caused by medical reasons, can be reversible or at least manageable if the underlying condition is treated (Mintzer and Brawman-Mintzer 1996). In fact, it has been stated that as many as 10% of elderly persons with dementia have a medically treatable condition causing the disorder (Stewart 1995).

3. **Agitation as an operant behavior.** This theoretical approach holds that agitated behaviors are learned responses influenced by either internal or external stimuli (Gugel 1994). Hunger and pain are among the most

frequently cited internal stimuli, but the physical and social environments that surround the person with dementia are the main external stimuli. Although patients with agitation syndromes are differentially affected by external stimuli, all agitated behaviors seem to increase when the elderly person with dementia is physically restrained, inactive, or alone (Cohen-Mansfield and Werner 1994; Werner et al. 1989). The underlying assumption of this conceptual framework is that the frequency, intensity, or duration of a given agitated behavior can be changed by systematically altering the internal or external stimuli.

4. **Agitation as an outcome of sensory deprivation.** Age-related changes in the functioning of the sensory systems, which are common among elderly persons (Krauss 1996), are exacerbated by the presence of dementia and can manifest themselves in the form of agitation. Researchers who use this conceptual framework base their understanding on the premise that increasing the sensory ability of the elderly agitated person (e.g., by using a hearing amplifier) can reduce the manifestation of the behavioral problems (Hay 1995).

Process Issues

Process issues relate to both the content and the operational aspects of nonpharmacological interventions in the treatment of agitated elderly persons.

Content Aspects

The range of nonpharmacological interventions described in the literature is extensive and diverse. Although an exhaustive description of these interventions is beyond the scope of this chapter, several thorough reviews have been published (e.g., Cohen-Mansfield and Werner 1994; Werner et al. 1995, on the management of verbally disruptive behaviors; and Cohen-Mansfield et al. 1996, on the management of wandering and aggressive behaviors).

Although most conceptual approaches are based on empirical knowledge about agitation and its correlates, few researchers have used this knowledge to develop specific hypotheses when designing nonpharmacological interventions and deciding which to implement. Only lately has the literature evolved in this area from descriptions of clinical interventions to more scientific evaluations of theoretically driven interventions (Cohen-Mansfield and Werner 1997, 1998; Denney 1997; Snyder et al. 1995). These efforts should be encouraged and expanded.

Generally, nonpharmacological interventions fall into four categories: nursing care adaptations, behavioral interventions, environmental changes, and sensory enhancement. The first three categories are based on the conceptualization of agitation as an operant behavior, and the last refers to agitation as the result of sensory deprivation.

Alterations in nursing care include enhancing the patient's physical comfort and fulfilling his or her basic physical needs (Nelson 1995) through symptom relief, assigning the same caregiver (Citrome and Green 1990; Travis and Moore 1991), breaking complex tasks into simple steps (Gerdner and Buckwalter 1994), and adopting a client-oriented care approach (Matthews et al. 1996).

Behavioral approaches include contingent reinforcement and time-outs (Baltes and Lascomb 1975; Rosberger and MacLean 1983; Vaccaro 1988a, 1988b). Environmental adaptations include use of environmental cues (e.g., two-dimensional grids to manage exit-seeking behaviors) (Chafetz 1990; Hussian and Brown 1987) and change of environmental structure (Negley and Manley 1990). Sensory stimulation interventions include the use of touch (Birchmore and Clague 1983; Mayers and Griffin 1990), activities (Cohen-Mansfield and Werner 1997; McGrowder-Lin and Bhatt 1988), and music (Cohen-Mansfield and Werner 1997; Ragneskog et al. 1996; Werner et al. 1995; Zachow 1984).

Lately, the implementation of multimodal interventions has been examined. One study (Rovner et al. 1996) described the implementation of a program combining activities, guidelines for the use of psychotropic medication, and educational rounds to reduce behavioral disorders in the nursing home. The use of a combination of approaches is also the basic assumption of special care units (Mintzer et al. 1993).

No discussion on nonpharmacological interventions can be complete without addressing two additional topics: caregiver training and the development of an individualized approach. Caregiver training must precede the implementation of any intervention because carrying out a management program requires time and a thorough understanding of the behavior under study (Vollen 1996). Without adequate knowledge and training on the part of the caregivers, not only may the intervention be unsuccessful, it may even increase the elderly person's agitation as well as the caregiver's stress and burden. Several educational programs for caregivers of nursing home residents have been described in the literature (Cohen-Mansfield et al. 1997; Feldt and Ryden 1992; Maxfield and Lewis 1995; Mentes and Ferraro 1989). No such studies, however, have been done in connection with informal caregivers.

In addition to generalized interventions, researchers should also include guidelines to tailor the intervention to the specific needs and characteristics of the elderly person. Our experience with the implementation of three behavioral interventions (i.e., one-to-one social interaction, the presentation of a videotape of a family member talking to the older person, and the use of music) for the management of verbally disruptive behaviors in nursing home residents shows that the effectiveness of the interventions was related to the specific type of verbally agitated behavior displayed (Cohen-Mansfield and Werner 1997). Another study (Tariot 1996) took this approach a step further, showing the importance of examining the association of different treatments with the type and stage of dementia, age at onset, duration of disease, and personality patterns (past and present).

Operational Aspects

A central issue in the development and implementation of nonpharmacological treatments is the elaboration of clear guidelines to the formal and informal caregivers (Reisberg 1996). The aim of these guidelines is twofold: they serve as a clear and detailed implementation protocol and allow replication by other researchers or with different subjects, thereby permitting evaluation of the protocol under varied circumstances. The guidelines must, however, allow the caregiver flexibility and creativity. If a management strategy is to be successful, it must be adapted not only to the characteristics and changing needs of the specific person but also to the characteristics of the caregiver and the institution.

Lately, several researchers have developed clinical decision trees to serve as guidelines in the implementation of nonpharmacological interventions (Chou et al. 1996; Mintzer and Brawman-Mintzer 1996; Potts et al. 1996). This technique offers an organized method for the development and assessment of behavioral interventions (White et al. 1996).

With minor variations, all researchers suggest the following steps in the implementation of nonpharmacological interventions for the management of agitation:

1. Performing a complete medical and neuropsychological evaluation to rule out any underlying medical or psychiatric conditions as well as polypharmacy problems.
2. Identifying the specific and measurable agitated behavior (i.e., defining which agitation factor is to be targeted for treatment).
3. Performing systematic observations of the events that occurred before and after the manifestation of the specific agitated behavior (i.e., determining both the antecedents and consequences of the disruptive behavior).

4. Systematically recording the type, frequency, and duration of the specific behavior before the implementation of any treatment.
5. Designing a treatment program specifically geared to the needs and characteristics of the elderly person, the caregiver, and the organization.
6. Implementing the treatment program.
7. Assessing and observing the effects of the intervention by recording the frequency and duration of the behavior during and after its implementation.

These steps form the basis for an ongoing cycle that must be repeated until the behavior has been successfully decreased.

Outcome Issues

Ultimately, the success of nonpharmacological interventions is measured by their effectiveness. The strongest evidence of effectiveness comes from well-designed controlled trials, yet relatively few have been conducted (Rovner et al. 1996). An alternative method is to establish the outcome criteria of effectiveness. The criteria suggested are 1) assessing the impact of nonpharmacological treatments on the quality of life of the elderly person and of the caregiver and 2) estimating the cost-effectiveness.

Elderly Person's Quality of Life

Quality of life for elderly persons with dementia has been defined as "personal competence in the physical and cognitive realms, absence of distress, presence of positive states, social engagement, and meaningful activity involvement" (Lawton 1996, p. 95). Assessing the effectiveness of nonpharmacological interventions requires judging whether their implementation has changed the elderly person's quality of life. Sometimes the change is reflected in the decrease of the targeted behavior itself, and sometimes it is seen in other aspects, such as the person's general mood, sleep patterns, or participation in structured activities. Presently, there is a dearth of information regarding the effect of nonpharmacological interventions on aspects of agitated persons' quality of life aside from the specific behavior under study.

Caregiver's Quality of Life

The effect of agitation on caregivers' quality of life has been well documented (Cohen-Mansfield 1996; Cohen-Mansfield and Werner 1994; Miller 1997). The manifestation of agitated behaviors has been associated with caregiver burnout, absenteeism, and turnover as well as with deterioration in physical and mental health (Chou et al. 1996). Assessing the effectiveness of nonpharmacological interventions requires an assessment of their effect not only on the elderly person, but also on the caregivers.

Assessing Cost Effectiveness

In making a final judgment about the outcome of nonpharmacological interventions, reliable information about their costs and benefits must be available. At times of cost containment, the decision to implement an intervention at the organizational level should be guided by such considerations. Few researchers, however, have assessed these issues. Rovner et al. (1996) assessed the cost-effectiveness of a multimodal intervention using a randomized, controlled trial design. Findings of this study showed neither cost reductions nor cost increments as a result of implementing the program. Mintzer et al. (1997) assessed the cost-effectiveness of a behavioral intensive care unit and found clear advantages, especially in the management of aggressive behaviors. Further research replicating and expanding these results is warranted.

Conclusions

In summary, as the number of elderly persons with dementia continues to increase, the nonpharmacological interventions aimed at reducing the manifestation of agitation pose a unique set of challenges to researchers and clinicians in the geriatric field. Although important advances have been noted in recent research, large gaps remain. In this chapter I have aimed to provide guidelines and thoughts for the development, implementation, and assessment of this important field.

References

Baltes MM, Lascomb SL: Creating a health institutional environment for the elderly via behavior management: the nurse as a change agent. Int J Nurs Stud 12:5–12, 1975

Birchmore T, Clague S: A behavioural approach to reduce shouting. Nurs Times 79:37–39, 1983

Carlson DL, Fleming KC, Smith GE, et al.: Management of dementia-related behavioral disturbances: a nonpharmacologic approach. Mayo Clin Proc 70:1108–1115, 1995

Chafetz PK: Two-dimensional grid is ineffective against demented patients' exiting through glass doors. Psychol Aging 5:146–147, 1990

Chou HW, Kaas MJ, Richie MF: Assaultive behavior in geriatric patients. J Gerontol Nurs 22:30–38, 1996

Citrome L, Green L: The dangerous agitated patient: what to do right now. Postgrad Med 87:231–236, 1990

Cohen-Mansfield J: New ways to approach manifestations of Alzheimer's disease and to reduce caregiver burden. Int Psychogeriatr 8(suppl):91–94, 1996

Cohen-Mansfield J, Billig N: Agitated behaviors in the elderly: a conceptual review. J Am Geriatr Soc 34:711–721, 1986

Cohen-Mansfield J, Werner P: Environmental influences on agitation: an integrative summary of an observational study. Am J Alzheimer Care Rel Disord Res 10:32–39, 1994

Cohen-Mansfield J, Werner P: Management of verbally disruptive behaviors in nursing home residents. J Gerontol: Biol Sci Med Sci 52(suppl A):369–377, 1997

Cohen-Mansfield J, Werner P: The effects of an enhanced environment on the behavior and mood of nursing home residents who pace. Gerontologist 38:199–208, 1998

Cohen-Mansfield J, Werner P, Marx MS, et al: Assessment and management of behavior problems in the nursing home, in Improving Care in the Nursing Home: Comprehensive Reviews of Clinical Research. Edited by Rubenstein LZ, Wieland D. Newbury Park, CA, Sage, 1993, pp 275–313

Cohen-Mansfield J, Marx MS, Werner P: Agitation in elderly persons: an integrative report of findings in a nursing home. Int Psychogeriatr 4:221–240, 1994

Cohen-Mansfield J, Werner P, Culppeper W, et al: Wandering and aggression, in The Practical Handbook of Clinical Gerontology. Edited by Carstensen LL, Edelstein BA, Dornbrand L. Thousand Oaks, CA, Sage, 1996, pp 374–397

Cohen-Mansfield J, Werner P, Culpepper J, et al: Evaluation of an in-service training program on dementia and wandering. J Gerontol Nurs 23:40–47, 1997

Denney A: Quiet music: an intervention for mealtime agitation? J Gerontol Nurs 23:16–23, 1997

Feldt KS, Ryden M: Aggressive behavior: educating nursing assistants. J Gerontol Nurs 18:3–12, 1992

Fleming KC, Evans JM: Pharmacologic therapies in dementia. Mayo Clin Proc 70:1116–1123, 1995

Franzen MD, Martin RC: Screening for neuropsychological impairment, in The Practical Handbook of Clinical Gerontology. Edited by Carstensen LL, Edelstein BA, Dornbrand L. Thousand Oaks, CA, Sage, 1996, pp 188–216

Gerdner L, Buckwalter K: A nursing challenge: assessment and management of agitation in Alzheimer's patients. J Gerontol Nurs April:11–20, 1994

Gugel RN: Behavioral approaches for managing patients with Alzheimer's disease and related disorders. Med Clin North Am 78:861–867, 1994

Hay D: Emerging perspectives in the treatment of behavioral and affective symptoms in Alzheimer's disease. Sixth Congress of the International Psychogeriatric Association. Berlin, Germany, 1995

Hussian RA, Brown DC: Use of two-dimensional grid patterns to treat hazardous ambulation in demented patients. J Gerontol 42: 558–560, 1987

Jeste DV, Krull AJ: Behavioral problems associated with dementia: diagnosis and treatment. Geriatrics 46:28–32, 1991

Krauss WS: Psychological perspectives on the normal aging process, in The Practical Handbook of Clinical Gerontology. Edited by Carstensen LL, Edelstein BA, Dornbrand L. Thousand Oaks, CA, Sage, 1996, pp 3–35

Kumar AM, Kumar M, Sevusg S, et al: Serotonin uptake and its kinetics in platelets of women with Alzheimer's disease. Psychiatry Res 59:145–150, 1995

Lawton MP: Behavioral problems and interventions in Alzheimer's disease: research needs. Int Psychogeriatr 8(suppl):95–98, 1996

Matthews EA, Farrell GA, Blackmore AM: Effects of an environmental manipulation emphasizing client-centred care on agitation and sleep in dementia sufferers in a nursing home. J Adv Nurs 24:439–447, 1996

Maxfield M, Lewis R: Creative methods for handling resistant behaviors of cognitively impaired elderly (abstract). Annual Scientific Meeting of the Gerontological Society of America, Los Angeles, CA, 1995

Mayers K, Griffin M: The play project: use of stimulus objects with demented patients. J Gerontol Nurs 16:32–37, 1990

McGrowder-Lin R, Bhatt A: A wanderer's lounge program for nursing home residents with Alzheimer's disease. Gerontologist 28: 607–609, 1988

Mentes JC, Ferraro J: Calming aggressive reactions: a preventive program. J Gerontol Nurs 15:22–27, 1989

Miller MF: Physically aggressive behavior during hygiene care. J Gerontol Nurs 23:24–39, 1997

Mintzer JE, Brawman-Mintzer O: Agitation as a possible expression of generalized anxiety disorder in demented elderly patients: toward a treatment approach. J Clin Psychiatry 57(suppl 7):55–63, 1996

Mintzer JE, Lewis L, Pennypacker L, et al: Behavioral intensive care unit (BICU): a new concept in the management of acute agitated behavior in elderly demented patients. Gerontologist 33:801–806, 1993

Mintzer JE, Colenda C, Waid LR, et al: Effectiveness of a continuum of care using brief and partial hospitalization for agitated dementia patients. Psychiatr Serv 48:1435–1439, 1997

Negley EN, Manley JY: Environmental interventions in assaultive behavior. J Gerontol Nurs 16:29–33, 1990

Nelson J: The influence of environmental factors in incidents of disruptive behavior. J Gerontol Nurs 21:19–24, 1995

Potts HW, Richie MF, Kaas MJ: Resistance to care. J Gerontol Nurs 22:11–16, 1996

Radebaugh TS, Buckholtz N, Khachaturian Z: Behavioral approaches to the treatment of Alzheimer's disease: research strategies. Int Psychogeriatr 8(suppl 1):7–12, 1996

Ragneskog H, Kilgren M, Karlsson I, et al: Dinner music for demented patients. Clin Nurs Res 5:262–282, 1996

Reisberg B: Behavioral intervention approaches to the treatment and management of Alzheimer's disease: a research agenda. Int Psychogeriatr 8(suppl):39–44, 1996

Rosberger Z, MacLean J: Behavioral assessment and treatment of "organic" behaviors in an institutionalized geriatric patient. Int J Behav Geriatr 1:33–46, 1983

Rovner BW, Steele CD, Shmueli Y, et al: A randomized trial of dementia care in nursing homes. J Am Geriatr Soc 44:7–13, 1996

Segal ES: Common medical problems in geriatric patients, in The Practical Handbook of Clinical Gerontology. Edited by Carstensen LL, Edelstein BA, Dornbrand L. Thousand Oaks, CA, Sage, 1996, pp 451–467

Sky AJ, Grossberg GT: The use of psychotropic medication in the management of problem behaviors in the patient with Alzheimer's disease. Med Clin North Am 78: 811–822, 1994

Snyder M, Egan EC, Burns KR: Interventions for decreasing agitation behaviors in persons with dementia. J Gerontol Nurs 21:34–40, 1995

Stewart JT: Management of behavior problems in the demented patient. Am Fam Physician 52:2311–2317, 1995

Tariot PN: Behavioral manifestations of dementia: a research agenda. Int Psychogeriatr 8(suppl):31–38, 1996

Travis S, Moore S: Nursing and medical care of primary dementia patients in a community hospital setting. Appl Nurs Res 4:14–18, 1991

Vaccaro FJ: Application of operant procedures in a group of institutionalized aggressive geriatric patients. Psychol Aging 3:22–28, 1988a

Vaccaro FJ: Successful operant conditioning procedures with an institutionalized aggressive geriatric patient. Int J Aging Hum Dev 26:71–79, 1988b

Vollen KH: Coping with difficult resident behaviors takes time. J Gerontol Nurs 22:22–26, 1996

Weinrich S, Egbert C, Eleazar GP, et al: Agitation: measurement, management, and intervention research. Arch Psychiatr Nurs 9:251–260, 1995

Werner P, Hay DP, Cohen-Mansfield J: Management of disruptive vocalizations in the nursing home. Nurs Home Med 3:217–225, 1995

Werner P, Cohen-Mansfield J, Braun J, et al: Physical restraints and agitation in nursing home residents. J Am Geriatr Soc 37:1122–1126, 1989

White MK, Kaas MJ, Richie MF: Vocally disruptive behavior. J Gerontol Nurs 22:23–29, 1996

Zachow KM: Helen, can you hear me? J Gerontol Nurs 10:18–22, 1984

CHAPTER 8

Psychotherapeutic Interventions

Leeanne Lott, M.S.W., L.C.S.W.
David T. Klein, Psy.D.

Agitation in patients with dementia not only affects the quality of life for both the patients and their caregivers but, according to Rabins et al. (1982), agitation is considered by most family caregivers to be their most serious problem. However, dementia per se does not explain the heterogeneity we see in the etiology and manifestation of agitated behaviors. In fact, agitation appears to involve a complex interaction of cognitive, affective, behavioral, interpersonal, and environmental components. Clinical interventions should address agitation's multifaceted nature.

Although pharmacological advances have significantly improved treatment strategies, agitation remains largely an issue of management. Psychotherapy is one intervention that has frequently been overlooked as an adjunctive means of helping patients with Alzheimer's disease (AD), family members, and professional staff manage agitation.

Psychotherapy has increasingly gained recognition as an important and effective treatment modality for many medical conditions. For example, the use of supplemental psychotherapy to improve outcomes in patients with chronic illnesses such as cancer and cardiac disease is well documented (Cottraux 1993; Grossarth-Maticek and Eysenck 1996; Spiegel 1995; Gabbard et al. 1997). Although the relationship between psychotherapy's curative factors and their impact on medical illness remains unclear, such interventions can be effectively used to maximize coping skills, address the emotional issues that inevitably accompany the disease, and reduce stress levels that tend to exacerbate the primary illness or produce psychiatric comorbidity. Despite the demonstrated efficacy of psychotherapeutic interventions in managing patients with chronic illnesses, however, there has been a paucity of systematic studies of such nonpharmacological treatment approaches to patients with AD.

Conceptual Overview of Psychotherapeutic Interventions in Alzheimer's Disease

Although there is no single empirically endorsed method of psychotherapy for use with this population, it is important to take a systemic stance with respect to treatment. That is, any successful intervention must address the patient, his or her caregiver (or caregivers), and relevant others, including additional family members, treating professionals, and, in the case of later-stage AD, nursing home staff. Whereas the methods of treatment for patients with AD comprise primarily cognitive-behavioral, environmental, educational, and supportive interventions, insight-oriented therapy is generally contraindicated for use in all but the most mildly demented patients. Caregivers often profit from learning about AD, training in behavioral management techniques, and attending to their own stress, including emotional issues that stem from the caregiving role. Hence, by definition, psychotherapeutic interventions generally involve a collaborative effort with the caregiver at a minimum, but optimally may include all individuals intimately involved in the care of the patient who has AD.

Like other chronic illnesses, AD is considered a "family illness" in the sense that it taxes the lives of all involved. Because of the demands associated with their role, caregivers frequently become increasingly isolated and unable to focus on their own needs, growth, and development (Goldstein 1996). They often present with symptoms of depression, anxiety, and somatization, and they are found to experience more psychiatric and health problems (Anthony et al. 1988; George and Gwyther 1986), visit their physicians more frequently, and take more medications than those without caregiving responsibilities (Brody 1989). Furthermore, as the disease progresses, the day-to-day worlds of patients with AD and their caregivers are often increasingly interwoven to the point that it becomes virtually impossible to treat an agitated patient without the cooperation and active involvement of the caregiver. Because of this highly involved and reciprocally influential relationship, caregiver mental health often suffers even more as a function of dementia-related behavioral disturbances such as agitation. For example, research has repeatedly indicated that such behavioral disturbances are highly predictive of caregiver psychological problems such as depression and anxiety (Brodaty 1996;

Donaldson et al. 1997; Victoroff et al. 1998). Interestingly, investigators have also found that patients with AD who are living with highly distressed caregivers tend to exhibit higher frequencies of behavioral problems, specifically agitation, than patients living with less distressed caregivers (Dunkin and Anderson-Hanley 1998). In combination, these findings empirically support the view that there is an interdependent and often sensitive psychological balance between patient and caregiver and emphasize the need to treat agitation systemically. Maximally effective psychotherapeutic interventions, therefore, need to address not only the patient and caregiver (or caregivers) but also the interpersonal and environmental context in which this relationship exists.

Assessment of Agitated Behaviors

If agitation is anything, it is complex. Although the literature has identified several of the common behavioral pathways that we now categorize as agitation, such as wandering and aggression (Cohen-Mansfield and Billig 1986), identifying and subsequently treating the cause of these behaviors remains considerably more elusive. One paradigm that is useful in understanding agitation is to go back to the basic explanation of behavior itself—namely, that behavior may be seen as the individual's attempt to actively adapt to his or her circumstances. In the case of an agitated patient with dementia, these attempts are made within the context of varying degrees of cognitive impairment that significantly interfere with the vital information feedback loop that the patient relies on to evaluate and adjust his or her behavior. In this sense, agitated behaviors may represent the patient's intentional or unintentional attempts to communicate needs, thoughts, and emotions through an increasingly taxed cognitive grasp on the world.

Furthermore, the circumstances affecting agitated behavior are multidetermined. In the case of patients with AD, three primary sets of variables may affect such circumstances. The first set consists of patient variables, including level of cognitive impairment, premorbid personality, psychological and physical needs or problems, and medications. Next are interpersonal variables, which essentially include the caregiver and close relations. The quality of these relationships with and styles of response to the patient with AD are two particularly influential factors in this category. The final set includes environmental variables such as the individual's familiarity and comfort with his or her surroundings as well as specific features of the environment, including the level of structure and stimulation. These three sets of variables are constantly changing and impinging on the

AD patient's increasingly taxed coping resources. Assessing the role played by each of these factors is the foundation of devising appropriate treatment strategies.

Often, a direct cause-and-effect relationship between these antecedent variables and agitated behaviors is not readily apparent. However, identifying patterns of agitated behaviors over time is a useful place to start the assessment process. This initial step serves to organize the caregiver's observations of the patient's behaviors. Although agitated behaviors may sometimes manifest for no apparent reason, a careful interview with the caregiver usually allows the clinician to identify clusters of agitated behaviors and begin to evaluate possible precipitants. A thorough interview should include an examination of the context in which the agitated behaviors occur and the interaction of the interpersonal, environmental, and patient-oriented variables. It is similarly important to assess and rule out antecedent conditions (e.g., pneumonia, urinary tract infections, delusions, hallucinations) that may be secondary to medical or psychiatric disorders. If such causes can be eliminated, it is best to begin addressing agitation with nonpharmacological interventions (Tariot 1996). The consensus among clinicians and researchers supports an individualized approach that focuses on environmental and psychotherapeutic interventions aimed at improving the quality of life for both the patient and his or her family members (Beck 1998). Furthermore, treatment algorithms have recently been developed to aid in clinical decision making for agitated patients with dementia (Pozuelo et al. 1998). Such advances in understanding have promoted better assessment, treatment planning, and intervention.

Designing Psychotherapeutic Interventions

As with other chronic illnesses, optimizing coping behavior serves as the cornerstone of psychotherapeutic work with agitated patients with dementia. This can be achieved through various interventions organized by the different levels at which the intervention is focused and by common behavioral problems in agitation and dementia.

Individuals with AD experience a cascade of losses of cognitive, functional, social, and psychological abilities. As such, reactions such as depression and anxiety are common, both of which not only cause great distress in their own right but may also exacerbate agitated behaviors in dementia. The primary goals of psychotherapeutic interventions in agitated patients with AD are to promote adjustment to these losses and optimize the individual's ability to cope with the emotional impact of the illness. This may be achieved through building or maintaining self-esteem, preserving integrity, and focusing and capitalizing on the patient's strengths. In the case of agitated patients with AD, the level of intervention is generally determined by the level of cognitive impairment and by the clinician's assessment of the patient's consequent capacity to profit from available interventions. With more mildly impaired patients, modified individual or group psychotherapy or supportive interventions may be implemented (Davies et al. 1995; Labarge and Trtanj 1995; Rentz 1995).

Working With Cognitively Impaired Individuals

Until more recently, it was widely assumed that cognitively impaired individuals would not benefit from individual psychotherapeutic interventions. However, with diagnosis increasingly occurring at an earlier stage, there has been added interest in intervention with this group. Studies indicate that cognitively impaired patients are capable of addressing difficult emotional issues (Miller 1989; Swanwick 1995) and may achieve significant benefits with individual psychotherapy, particularly when the approach is structured and the goals are well defined (Cohen 1989; Sadavoy and Robinson 1989). Although efficacy has not yet been firmly established, there have been reports of improvement in depressive symptoms (Swanwick 1995). Furthermore, Jeste and Krull (1991) indicated that patients with mild dementia were able to make progress in coming to terms with their deficits and adjusting to their situations.

Various psychotherapeutic approaches have been used and studied with older adults, including cognitive, behavioral, psychodynamic, supportive, psychoeducational, and reminiscence (Teri and Logsdon 1992; Teri and McCurry 1994). Research on cognitive-behavioral therapy with this group has been the most extensive, demonstrating this intervention to be particularly effective in the treatment of depression. Moreover, a few of the studies that have extended the treatment to individuals with AD, caregivers, and older adults residing in long-term care facilities have had positive outcomes (Thompson and Gallagher 1984, 1985, 1986; Thompson et al. 1987, 1991b). Empirical evidence supports the effectiveness of the other interventions as well (Gallagher and Thompson 1982). Specifically, they have been shown to decrease depressed mood, improve life satisfaction, and bolster self-esteem in older adults (Mintzer et al. 1998). One study comparing the efficacy of three of the approaches (cognitive, behavioral, and psychodynamic) in the treatment of depressed older adults found the interventions to be equally effective, with an overall response rate of 70% (Thompson et al. 1987). Moreover, efficacy has been equal or superior to treatment with medication (Thompson et al. 1991a).

Gallagher and Thompson (1991) recommended numerous modifications to the cognitive approach to address the special problems of older adults. They suggested initially preparing the patient for therapy by discussing in advance what is involved. For example, the therapist might describe therapy as the process of learning techniques to better deal with stress and loss and encourage the patient's active participation. They also recommended strengthening the older adult's learning capacity by addressing any reluctance to try new suggestions. Added attention should be given to the process of termination by terminating therapy more slowly, gradually reducing the frequency of sessions, discussing the potential for future problems, and encouraging the patient to return when needed.

Thompson et al. (1999b) provided further modifications, suggesting that therapists should strive to be especially flexible, take a more active role, encourage a focus on the here and now, generally advance more slowly, and use the patient's language as much as possible. When working with patients with cognitive changes or sensory deficits, the authors also suggest that key points of sessions be presented in several modalities. For example, the therapist may review important themes throughout sessions, encourage note taking, tape sessions for the patient to review, and assign exercises for the patient to complete between sessions (Thompson et al. 1991b).

Life review and reminiscence, which theoretically help individuals to put past experiences in perspective and process unresolved conflicts (Butler 1963), continue to be popular approaches for intervening with cognitively intact as well as impaired older adults in both individual and group settings. Because these approaches rely on long-term memories, which are typically better preserved than short-term information in cognitively impaired individuals, they may be particularly appropriate for this group. Reminiscence and life review not only capitalize on the strengths of cognitively impaired older adults but are also easily implemented. Although primarily anecdotal, results are generally positive. Older adults commonly find reminiscing to be a pleasant, comfortable activity that can reduce feelings of resistance and fear while simultaneously promoting feelings of competence and control (Swanwick 1995). One study of 27 nursing home residents with AD reported significant improvement in self-reported mood compared with residents participating in supportive and control groups (Goldwasser 1987). It is important to note, however, that for more impaired or psychotic patients, this approach is less effective than more structured, less verbally oriented approaches. Furthermore, it can result in a worsening of agitation or behavioral disturbance (Lesser et al. 1981).

The range of goals and objectives that may be addressed with cognitively impaired individuals through the use of psychotherapy is broad, and selection depends on the particular patient's needs, problems, and abilities. Support and assistance are commonly provided to help individuals with mild dementia accept their diagnoses, cope with declining abilities, and adjust to their environments. More specific goals may include establishing rapport and understanding to reduce feelings of loneliness and isolation; supporting positive reminiscing to encourage feelings of competence and worth; and minimizing excess disability (including addressing sensory deficits, medical problems, and concomitant psychiatric disorders such as depression and psychosis) as well as decreasing isolation, withdrawal, and inactivity (Brody et al. 1971). Additionally, individuals may be guided toward focusing on activities, interests, and abilities that continue to provide satisfaction and a positive sense of self-worth. Assistance with decision making and long-term planning may be provided as well.

Working With the Family

Although psychotherapy with cognitively impaired individuals is beginning to receive more attention, the primary focus of intervention has traditionally been the family. Zarit and Teri (1991) summarized the empirical research on psychotherapy with family caregivers in their extensive review. Both individual and group treatment have been shown to be effective, with reductions in anxiety and depression as well as improvement in self-reports of caregiver distress and burden. In addition, studies have demonstrated that such interventions can lead to significant improvements in behavioral problems of impaired patients that are being cared for as well as to delays in nursing home placement (Greene and Monahan 1989; Pinkston and Linsk 1984).

Education About the Disease

One of the most critical functions clinicians can perform is educating patients' families about AD and its effects. Providing an appreciation for the range of agitated behaviors associated with dementia may assist with planning and allow caregivers to prepare themselves for handling behaviors that may arise. Because family members frequently have expectations that are no longer realistic or make attributions that are inappropriate or incorrect, they may also need to learn how to anticipate and more appropriately interpret agitated behaviors (Roper et al. 1991). For example, a patient who continually asks: "When are we going to get there?" while riding in the car may lead the family member driving to question whether the patient is deliberately trying to get on his or her nerves or even criticizing the speed of the driving. By stressing that repeated questions are a result of the patient's inability to remember what he has previously asked and a symptom of the illness beyond his control, the family member may feel less anger toward the patient and less overall stress. Family members may also inappropriately personalize the patient's behaviors. They may complain, for example, "If he really loved me, he wouldn't expect me to wait on him hand and foot" or "She must be mad at me, because she didn't do anything for my birthday." Moreover, family members frequently assume that the patient is still capable of making important decisions and controlling or changing his or her behavior. For example, family members might assume that a patient "just doesn't seem to care about her appearance anymore," when in fact the patient is losing her ability to groom and dress independently or is not able to remember the last time she bathed.

Stress of Caregiving

Another key area for intervention is family members' ability to provide care and cope with an individual who has dementia. Family members may benefit from education about the prevalence of stress among caregivers and the impact that stress can have on both caregiver and patient. In addition to the deleterious effects on the caregiver's mental and physical health already discussed, there is evidence that caregiver stress has a negative impact on the care provided. Therefore, the importance of caring for the caregiver should be given particular emphasis, and the range of options for getting support and assistance should be explored. Therapists may strongly urge increased involvement of other family members when possible and facilitate setting up a meeting with family members early in the disease process to discuss how each can contribute to the patient's care. In addition, involvement in support groups should be encouraged to provide additional opportunities for family members to share feelings and experiences, learn, and gain support from their peers. Formal and informal options for providing respite care, including in-home care, adult day care, and short-term respite care, may also be reviewed and explored. The value of regular respite in preventing caregiver stress and burden should be emphasized. Family members also frequently benefit from additional assistance with the practical aspects of selecting and arranging care, including how to decide which care option best meets their needs and how to evaluate professional caregivers and facilities.

It is critical to keep in mind that the focus of the intervention efforts may change over the course of the patient's illness. Early on, family members may be wrestling with accepting the diagnosis. In addition, knowing what to expect for the future, including financial and legal considerations, may be a key concern. As the illness progresses, increasing care needs, behavioral problems, and issues of safety become more salient. Caregivers may also need more assistance dealing with feelings of burden and loss. During later stages, issues of placement and management in a long-term care facility, feelings of guilt and loneliness, and advance directives may be addressed in more depth.

Communication

Communication is another crucial area that should be addressed with families. Most importantly, family members should be provided with education, support, and assistance to allow them to gradually adapt their communication style as the patient's dementia progresses. Several essential facets of communication should be targeted. With the dementing individual's increasing impairment, the use of logic and rationality become increasingly ineffectual. Consequently, deeply ingrained habits and communication patterns such as explaining, reasoning, and arguing not only lose their effectiveness but can also lead to increases in agitation and behavioral disturbances. As an alternative, the patient's family should be encouraged to address and provide support for underlying emotions the patient may be experiencing (Feil 1993). Family members should also be instructed in the use of distraction, which can be used in combination with other techniques or as an effective alternative, particularly when other strategies are not working. A patient who is becoming increasingly agitated with efforts at trying to get him to leave for a doctor's appointment may cooperate if a family member states in a soothing manner: "I understand it can be stressful and scary to go to the doctor. But you don't have to worry because I'll stay with you. I love you and want to help you stay calm and healthy." If, however, the patient continues to resist, the family member might use distraction, shifting the focus to getting a drink of water before they leave or having lunch after the appointment.

As the dementia progresses, family members may benefit from further support, modeling, and role playing to help them simplify their communication by using shorter, uncomplicated sentences and simpler words. With increasing deterioration in comprehension, family members and caregivers should be encouraged to restate their sentence using the exact same words when the demented individual doesn't appear to understand. Similarly, as verbal expression skills diminish, families may be counseled on the appropriateness of filling in words or phrases when the patient is experiencing word-finding difficulty. These techniques can be useful in decreasing stress for the patient who is prone to agitation as well as for his or her family members.

Finally, family members should be educated about the increased role of nonverbal communication when relating to patients with dementia (Knopman and Sawyer-DeMaris 1990). The importance of caregivers attending to their tone of voice and stance, which become more salient as patients are increasingly unable to fully comprehend the verbal content of what is said, should be addressed. For example, one patient with dementia frequently became agitated when her husband arrived to pick her up from an adult day care facility. After exploration, the husband began to recognize that he was typically tense and impatient after rushing to pick up his wife after a difficult day at the office. With increased awareness, he was able to use relaxation techniques to help him feel more calm and relaxed when he began to note symptoms of stress. As a result, his wife's agitation diminished significantly during the transition from day care to home.

Assistance With Medication Treatment and Monitoring

Psychotherapy may assist in facilitating treatment with medications as well as in monitoring efficacy and side effects. Because therapists sometimes have more frequent and intimate contact with family members than do other health care providers, they are in a key position to provide education about the availability and usefulness of medications in the treatment of agitation. In addition, clinicians may need to address family biases toward medication that can adversely affect the patient's treatment. For example, some family members want to try medication immediately without first attempting to alter communication strategies, the patient's daily routine, or the environment. Conversely, other families with negative attitudes about medications may be hesitant to even consider them as an option despite the potential for harm to the patient or others posed by the agitated behavior. Both types of families may benefit from guidance to help them accept when treatment with medication may be the most appropriate choice. Assistance in monitoring compliance and the efficacy of treatment may be a focus of the intervention as well.

Many family members also benefit from support in working with the patient's physician and treatment team. The clinician is able to encourage the family to remain actively involved with the physician or treatment team and assist the family in communicating the patient's symptoms and needs. Some family members may also need additional problem-solving and skill development to help them achieve these goals. For example, one husband who repeatedly became flustered by the time constraints and other situational demands of accompanying his wife to the doctor learned through the process of problem solving to make a list before the appointment of the topics he wanted to address with the physician. This led to a decrease in the husband's stress and optimized the medical care his wife was receiving through better communication of her problems and needs.

Environmental Approaches

Educating and assisting family members and caregivers about the role of environmental modifications in decreasing agitation and the frequency of catastrophic reactions should be another focus of psychotherapy. In general, the goals of preserving or increasing familiarity, structure, predictability, and safety while minimizing noise and distractions should be emphasized. Furthermore, it is frequently recommended that colors in the environment should be soft and calming and that all clutter should be removed. Soothing music may be suggested because of its beneficial effects; the constant noise of television and radio are discouraged because of its potential to be disturbing for persons with dementia. Similarly, loud noises such as doorbells, telephone rings, and alarms may need to be modified or eliminated.

Keeping in mind the individual differences in levels of tolerance among cognitively impaired individuals, it is important to address with family members other key aspects of the environment, including activities and socializing. Although a regular routine is encouraged and activities and socializing may provide beneficial stimulation, too much stimulation may lead to increased agitation and behavioral disturbances. In general, these adverse emotional and behavioral reactions may be minimized by limiting the number of unfamiliar social contacts. However, it is also important to consider the intensity of interactions. For example, it is well known that a screaming, agitated patient in a nursing home leads to increases in the level of agitation among exposed fellow residents. In addition, the shouting and physical play of children can be misinterpreted and lead to agitation and even physical aggressiveness. In conclusion, it is important to provide a level of stimulation geared to the individual patient's needs and capabilities.

Interventions for Specific Agitated Behaviors

Psychotherapeutic interventions may focus on helping family members deal with specific behavioral problems, including pacing and wandering, screaming, sundowning, and insomnia. Goals may include helping to assess the problem behaviors in depth, including the frequency, duration, and timing of the behavior; providing education about the various approaches that may be used to deal with a given problem; assisting in the implementation of the approach; monitoring the efficacy of the strategy chosen; and problem solving as needed to ensure consistency.

Pacing and Wandering

Psychotherapeutic interventions may serve to help family and caregivers identify the causes of pacing and wandering behaviors in the individual with dementia as well as provide education and training in the various strategies that have been found to be helpful in managing or limiting these behaviors. A thorough assessment of the problem behavior is the first step to intervention. Because akathisia is a side effect of some medications, this possibility should be ruled out as well. For many other individuals with dementia, wandering is associated with self-stimulation or attempts to leave. Family members may be taught behavioral and environmental modification strategies and skills that can be used to manage this behavior. For example, patients may wear identification bracelets, simple stop signs or other devices may be used as barriers, and complex or strategically placed locks may be installed on doors.

Screaming

Family members and caregivers may be educated about the potential causes of as well as the range of strategies used to address this particularly distressful behavior. Again, it is critical to emphasize that the initial step should be a thorough assessment of the behavior to determine whether medical, psychiatric, or environmental factors may be contributing. Research indicates that screaming and other disruptive vocalizing can be associated with pain and that these behaviors frequently resolve with adequate medical treatment. These behaviors may also be features of an atypical depression that often responds to treatment with antidepressant agents.

Screaming is also a common response to the provision of personal-care activities such as grooming, bathing, and toileting. In these instances, caregivers may be counseled to first try different strategies in approaching and communicating with the patient. The use of music is widely suggested and has been noted to be particularly helpful to soothe as well as to provide stimulation to patients who are socially isolated. Another approach involves using behavioral strategies and rewarding patients for desirable behavior while simultaneously ignoring screaming and other disruptive vocalizations. A newer strategy that is receiving increased attention involves the use of a hearing augmenter, a device that amplifies sound. The augmenter serves to amplify the sounds of the patient's vocalizations, which is unpleasant for the patient and thereby discourages the behavior.

Sundowning and Disruptions in the Sleep Cycle

The appearance or worsening of symptoms in the late afternoon or early evening, referred to as *sundowning,* is a common complaint among family caregivers and nursing home staff. However, there has been significant disagreement in the literature regarding not only the etiology of the syndrome but whether it even exists (Cohen-Mansfield et al. 1989; Duggan and McDonald 1992; Evans 1987). Regardless of the controversy, recommended management strategies are similar to those directed at improving sleep. As with other symptoms of agitation, physical pain or illness should first be ruled out. Efforts may then be directed toward education and problem solving to assist with improving sleep hygiene. Because normal age-related changes in sleep are exaggerated in patients with AD, patients, families, and other caregivers frequently have an inadequate understanding of and unrealistic expectations regarding sleep. Consequently, simply providing education that addresses these beliefs and expectations may lead to significant reductions in stress (Winograd and Jarvik 1986). In addition, intervention may involve providing specific suggestions and problem solving to improve sleep hygiene. Suggestions may include promoting daytime structure, socializing, activities, and exercise; avoiding caffeine, alcohol, and daytime napping; and eliminating loud noises, bright lights, extreme temperatures, and other stimuli that may disrupt sleep (Gillin and Byerley 1990; Okawa et al. 1991; Swanwick 1995; Swanwick and Clare 1991).

Conclusions

Psychotherapy can be a useful intervention in the treatment of agitation in older adults with dementia. Various approaches may be used, including cognitive, behavioral, psychodynamic, and reminiscence. Empirical studies have demonstrated the effectiveness of these interventions with the elderly, with response rates of 70% and reports of improvement equaling that achieved by treatment with medication. Psychotherapeutic interventions may be used with patients as well as family members and caregivers and applied to a wide range of goals. In this chapter we have reviewed the basis for taking a systemic approach, treating both the patient and care-giver; outlined various psychotherapy approaches; and reviewed related research. We have discussed some goals to consider and provided recommendations for issues to be addressed with family members. Finally, we have made suggestions for using psychotherapy to deal with specific behavioral manifestations of agitation.

References

Anthony CR, Zarit SH, Gatz M: Symptoms of psychological distress among caregivers of dementia patients. Psychol Aging 3:225–248, 1988

Beck CK: Psychosocial and behavioral interventions for Alzheimer's disease patients and their families. Am J Ger Psychiatry 6(suppl):41–48, 1998

Brodaty H: Caregivers and behavioral disturbances: effects and interventions. Int Psychogeriatr 8(suppl 3):455–458, 1996

Brody EM: Family at risk, in Alzheimer's Disease: Treatment and Family Stress (DHHS Publ No [ADM] 89-1569). Edited by Light E, Lebowitz B. Rockville, MD, National Institute of Mental Health, 1989, pp 2–49

Brody E, Kleban MH, Lawton MP, et al: Excess disabilities of mentally impaired aged: impact of individualized treatment. Gerontologist 11:133, 1971

Butler RN: The life review: an interpretation of reminiscence in the aged. Psychiatry 26:65–76, 1963

Cohen GD: Psychodynamic perspectives in the clinical approach to brain disease in the elderly, in Psychiatric Consequences of Brain Disease in the Elderly. Edited by Conn D, Grek A, Sadavoy J. New York, Plenum, 1989, pp 85–99

Cohen-Mansfield J, Billig N: Agitated behaviors in the elderly: a conceptual review. J Am Geriatr Soc 34:711–721, 1986

Cohen-Mansfield J, Watson V, Meade W: Does sundowning occur in residents of an Alzheimer's unit? Int J Geriatr Psychiatry 4:293–298, 1989

Cottraux J: Behavioral psychotherapy applications in the medically ill. Psychother Psychosom 60:119–128, 1993

Davies HD, Robinson D, Bevill L: Supportive group experience for patients with early-stage Alzheimer's disease. J Am Geriatr Soc 43:1068–1069, 1995

Donaldson C, Tarrier N, Burns A: The impact of symptoms on dementia caregivers. Br J Psychiatry 170:62–68, 1997

Duggan K, McDonald C: Wandering and twilight in a female psycho-geriatric population. Psychiatr Bull 16:479–481, 1992

Dunkin JJ, Anderson-Hanley C: Dementia caregiver burden: a review of the literature and guidelines for assessment and intervention. Neurology 51(suppl 1):53–60, 1998

Evans LK: Sundown syndrome in the institutionalized elderly. J Am Geriatr Soc 35:101–108, 1987

Feil N: The Validation Breakthrough. Baltimore, MD, Health Professionals Press, 1993

Gabbard GO, Lazar SG, Hornberger JM, et al: The economic impact of psychotherapy: a review. Am J Psychiatry 154(2):147–155, 1997

Gallagher DE, Thompson LW: Depression in the Elderly: A Behavioral Treatment Manual. Los Angeles, CA, University of Southern California Press, 1981

Gallagher DE, Thompson LW: Differential effectiveness of psychotherapies for the treatment of major depressive disorders in older adult patients. Psychotherapy: Theory, Research, and Practice 19:482–491, 1982

George LK, Gwyther LP: Caregiver well-being: a multidimensional examination of family caregivers of demented adults. Gerontologist 26:253–259, 1986

Gillin JC, Byerley WF: The diagnosis and management of insomnia. N Engl J Med 322:239–248, 1990

Goldstein MZ: Families of older adults, in Comprehensive Review of Geriatric Psychiatry, 2nd Edition. Washington, DC, American Psychiatric Press, 1996, pp 881–906

Goldwasser AN, Averbach SM, Harkins SW: Cognitive, affective, and behavioral effects of reminiscence group therapy on demented elderly. Int J Aging Hum Dev 25:209–222, 1987

Greene VL, Monahan DJ: The effect of a support and educational program on stress and burden among family caregivers to frail elderly persons. Gerontologist 29:472–477, 1989

Grossarth-Maticek R, Eysenck HJ: Psychological factors in the treatment of cancer and coronary heart disease, in The Hatherleigh Guide to Issues in Modern Therapy. New York, Hatherleigh Press, 1996, pp 53–68

Jeste DV, Krull AJ: Behavioral problems associated with dementia: diagnosis and treatment. Geriatrics 46:28–34, 1991

Knopman DS, Sawyer-DeMaris S: Practical approach to managing behavioral problems in dementia patients. Geriatrics 45:27–35, 1990

Labarge E, Trtanj F: A support group for people in the early stages of dementia of the Alzheimer type. Special issue: community-based programs and services for aging and special care populations. J App Geriatr 14:289–301, 1995

Lesser J, Lazarus LW, Frankel R, et al: Reminiscence group therapy with psychotic geriatric inpatients. Gerontologist 21:291–296, 1981

Miller MD: Opportunities for psychotherapy in the management of dementia. J Geriatr Psychiatry Neurol 2:11–17, 1989

Mintzer JE, Hoernig NHA, Mirski DF: Treatment of agitation in patients with dementia. Clin Geriatr Med 14:1457–1475, 1998

Okawa M, Mishima K, Hishikawa Y, et al: Circadian rhythm disorders in sleep-waking and body temperature in elderly patients with dementia and their treatment. Sleep 14:478–485, 1991

Pinkston EM, Linsk NL: Behavioral family intervention with the impaired elder. Gerontologist 26:576–583, 1984

Pozuelo L, Franco K, Palmer R: Agitated dementia: drug vs no drug. Cleveland Clinic Journal of Medicine 65:191–199, 1998

Rabins PV, Mace NL, Lucas MJ: The impact of dementia in the family. JAMA 248:333–335, 1982

Rentz CA: Reminiscence: a supportive intervention for the person with Alzheimer's disease. J Psychosoc Nurs Ment Health Serv 33:15–20, 1995

Roper JM, Shapira J, Chang BL: Agitation in the demented patient: a framework for management. J Gerontol Nurs 17:17–21, 1991

Sadavoy J, Robinson A: Psychotherapy and the cognitively impaired elderly, in Psychiatric Consequences of Brain Disease in the Elderly. Edited by Conn D, Brek A, Sadavoy J. New York, Plenum, 1989, pp 101–135

Spiegel D: Essentials of psychotherapeutic intervention for cancer patients. Support Care Cancer 3:252–256, 1995

Swanwick GRJ: Nonpharmacological treatment of behavioral symptoms, in Behavioral Complications in Alzheimer's Disease. Edited by Lawlor, BA. Washington, DC, American Psychiatric Press, 1995, pp 183–207

Swanwick GRJ, Clare AW: The management of insomnia. Journal of the Irish Colleges of Physicians and Surgeons 20:249–250, 1991

Tariot PN: Treatment strategies for agitation and psychosis in dementia. J Clin Psychiatry 57(suppl 14):21–29, 1996

Teri L, Logsdon RG: The future of psychotherapy with older adults. Psychotherapy 29:81–87,1992

Teri L, McCurry SM: Psychological therapies, in Textbook of Geriatric Neuropsychiatry. Edited by Coffey CD, Cummings JL. Washington, DC, American Psychiatric Press, 1994, pp 662–682

Thompson LW, Gallagher D: Efficacy of psychotherapy in the treatment of late-life depression. Adv Behav Res Ther 6:127–139, 1984

Thompson LW, Gallagher D: Depression and its treatment in the elderly. Aging 348:14–18, 1985

Thompson LW, Gallagher D: Psychotherapy for late-life depression. Generations 10:38–41, 1986

Thompson LW, Gallagher D, Breckenridge JS: Comparative effectiveness of psychotherapies for depressed elders. J Consult Clin Psychol 55:385–390, 1987

Thompson LW, Gallagher-Thompson D, Hanser S, et al: Treatment of late-life depressions with cognitive/behavioral therapy or desipramine. Poster presented at the annual meeting of the American Psychological Association, San Francisco, CA, August 1991a

Thompson LW, Gantz F, Florsheim M, et al: Cognitive-behavioral therapy in affective disorders in the elderly, in New Techniques in the Psychotherapy of Older Patients. Edited by Myers WA. Washington, DC, American Psychiatric Press, 1991b, pp 3–19

Victoroff J, Mack WJ, Nielson KA: Psychiatric complications of dementia: impact on caregivers. Dementia and Geriatric Cognitive Disorders 9:50–55, 1998

Winograd CH, Jarvik LF: Physician management of the demented patient. J Am Geriatr Soc 34:295–308, 1986

Zarit SH, Teri L: Interventions and services for family caregivers. Annu Rev Gerontol Geriatr 11:241–265, 1991

CHAPTER 9

Bright Light Therapy

Andrew Satlin, M.D.
David Harper, Ph.D.
Yvette Rheaume, R.N.
Ladislav Volicer, M.D., Ph.D.

In this chapter, the term *bright light therapy* refers to the practice of exposing patients with dementia to periods of illumination greater than that ordinarily encountered indoors, for the specific purpose of treating behavioral disorders. The potential benefits in institutional settings of bright, constant, ordinary indoor illumination during the day or low levels of light at night to aid visual discrimination, improve orientation, and reduce illusions is not discussed here. These practices are common sense, and despite the lack of rigorous research findings to support them, they should be followed in all nursing homes. Bright light therapy, on the other hand, is a relatively new and still experimental procedure. Readers are cautioned at the outset that this chapter does not provide clear, clinical recommendations for the use of bright light therapy that are practical for all clinicians treating patients with dementia because of the absence of adequate data on which to base such recommendations. Instead, more attention is given to the theoretical basis for research into the usefulness of such therapy and the findings and limitations from the few studies that have been published. It is hoped that this background information and the summary and conclusions that follow will be helpful to practicing clinicians who evaluate the research literature that will be published in the next few years and that may soon result in more useful clinical guidelines.

Background: The Concept of Sundowning

The origin of the term *sundowning* is buried in clinical lore, but today the term is most commonly used to refer to a syndrome of recurring confusion and increased agitation in patients with dementia occurring the late afternoon or early evening. In the community, sundowning is often said to occur when a patient with dementia does not sleep after going to bed but instead wanders around the house, attempts to leave, and shouts or becomes aggressive in response to attempts at redirection. In institutional settings, increased restlessness and vocalization are often observed around the time of the afternoon change of nursing shift. The suspected association between agitation and reduced ambient light that the term *sundowning* suggests was the basis for Cameron's 1941 experiment to elicit such behaviors (Cameron 1941). In that uncontrolled study, elderly patients with memory disturbances who developed delirium and agitation soon after going to bed at night were put in a dark room earlier in the day. In every instance, delirium appeared within 1 hour after the patient had been put in the dark room; in some cases, agitation also developed. Symptoms resolved within an hour of the lights' being turned back on. The appearance of delirium was earlier and more marked in patients in whom it was most severe at night.

Despite anecdotal observations such as these, it is not entirely clear that the sundowning pattern of agitation represents a distinct clinical entity with its own pathophysiology and risk factors. Research on the prevalence and correlates of this syndrome has been hampered by the lack of operationalized criteria for diagnosis. In one study, disturbed behaviors in nursing home patients were rated by research assistants during 10-minute portions of a 2-hour period in the morning and afternoon for 2 consecutive days, and sundowning was diagnosed if the mean afternoon score exceeded the morning score (Evans 1987). By this definition, 11 of 89 patients (12%) could have been classified as sundowners.

In another study, trained observers recorded the number of times that agitated behaviors occurred during a 3-minute period for each hour of the 24-hour day over a 2-month span (Cohen-Mansfield et al. 1989). The total number of behaviors recorded during the hours from 6 A.M. to 3 P.M. was compared with the number recorded from 3 P.M. to 11 P.M. Two of the eight residents were considered sundowners, but four others had more agitation in the earlier part of the day.

A third study defined sundowning based on global assessments by nursing staff of patients' behavior over a 3-week period (Little et al. 1995). Patients were classified as sundowners if all three nurse raters thought

that they manifested the appearance or exacerbation of behavioral disturbances associated with the afternoon or evening hours (or both). Other patients were classified as probable sundowners if identified by two of the
three nurse raters and as possible sundowners if identified by one of the
nurses. By these criteria, 10% of 71 patients with severe dementia and Alzheimer's disease (AD) were sundowners, with an additional 14% probable
sundowners and 21% possible sundowners. The results from these three
studies suggest that only 10%–25% of inpatients with moderate to severe
dementia manifest a behavioral pattern of agitation consistent with the
concept of sundowning. Nevertheless, the identification of sundowning in
studies with varying methodology is strong evidence in favor of the existence of such a temporal pattern, at least in a subgroup of patients with dementia.

Is Sundowning Related to Sleep Disorders?

The risk factors associated with sundowning are poorly established. One
study found associations between sundowning in nursing home residents
and the presence of dementia, more severe cognitive impairment, incontinence, more recent admission to the facility, room transfer within the previous month, and fewer medical diagnoses (Evans 1987), but another
study found no association with degree of cognitive impairment or medical diagnoses (Little et al. 1995). More substantial evidence favors an association between sundowning and the presence of sleep disorders. Studies
in patients with AD suggest that sleep–wake patterns become progressively more disrupted as the severity of dementia increases (Ancoli-Israel
et al. 1989; Prinz et al. 1982a, 1982b; Vitiello et al. 1990). Clinical changes
can best be described as fragmentation of sleep, with increased awakening
at night, more time spent awake at night, greater amounts of daytime
sleep, and more transitions from sleep to wakefulness even during naps.
Among demented patients with these sleep disturbances, daytime agitation is more common (Cohen-Mansfield and Marx 1990; Rebok et al. 1991).

The mechanism underlying an association between sundowning and
sleep disturbance in patients with dementia is not known. Several hypotheses have been proposed, some of which have experimental support. One
possibility is that the agitation and confusion of sundowning are caused by
the disorientation that accompanies awakening from sleep, especially when
this awakening occurs in an environment that is deficient in orienting cues,
such as a darkened or unfamiliar room. This hypothesis would, of course,
explain the frequency of sundowning in patients with dementia, who experience more awakenings from sleep during the day and whose cognitive

impairment renders them more susceptible to disorientation in any environment. In support of this hypothesis, patients who are more likely to be awakened by nursing staff during the night exhibit more sundowning or aggressive behavior (Cohen-Mansfield and Marx 1990; Evans 1987).

In an early study, some patients with DSM-II–defined (American Psychiatric Association 1968) chronic brain syndrome appeared to awaken repeatedly from rapid eye movement (REM) sleep into a delirious activated state with delusional ideas (Feinberg et al. 1967). Patients are more likely to awaken with agitation after sunset than during daytime hours, suggesting that some of the nocturnal confusion seen in patients with dementia may be caused by the effects of awakening from sleep into darkness (Bliwise et al. 1993). Thus, the combination of an increased tendency to daytime sleep, decreased ability to maintain a sleeping state, and the effects of awakening from REM sleep may result in sundowning and explain its association with sleep disturbance.

Sundowning and Sleep Disturbance: Disorders of Circadian Rhythms?

Another possible explanation for the association of sundowning and sleep disturbance is that both represent manifestations of an underlying dysfunction in the brain's circadian timekeeping system. Human circadian (approximately 24-hour) rhythms are necessary for the successful adaptation of both behavioral and physiological processes to changes occurring in the environment. Sundowning and sleep disturbances are both characterized by inappropriately timed and modulated rest and activity. Both also have clinical features in common with other syndromes believed to involve dysregulation of circadian rhythmicity, such as dyssomnias, affective illness (particularly seasonal affective disorder [SAD]), "jet lag," and intolerance to shift work (Czeisler et al. 1987; Lewy et al. 1987; Souetre et al. 1989).

Formal chronobiological studies lend some support to the hypothesis that the pathophysiology of AD may include disruption of normal circadian rhythms. Abnormalities of endocrine and enzyme level rhythms and of the phasic architecture of sleep have been found in patients with AD (Cornelissen et al. 1985; Loewenstein et al. 1982; Prinz et al. 1982a; Touitou et al. 1982; Vitiello et al. 1992). Several studies have used electronic monitors to record the levels and patterns of locomotor activity in patients with dementia over periods of several days. The raw activity data are then transformed mathematically to generate variables indicative of circadian rhythmicity. These variables include the percentage of total daily activity occurring during the night (percent nocturnal activity); interdaily stability, a measure that may reflect the degree of coupling of the activity rhythm to environmental timing cues; and interdaily variability, which may reflect daytime naps or nighttime arousals. A simultaneous nonlinear least-squares cosinor curve-fitting analysis of the raw activity data can also be used to calculate the mean activity level, the amplitude of the circadian rhythm (a measure of its strength and stability), and its acrophase (the clock time of peak activity). Although results from such studies have been variable, findings have included lower interdaily stability, higher intra-daily variability, higher percentage of nocturnal activity, lower rhythm amplitudes, and delayed acrophases in mid- to late-stage institutionalized patients with AD compared with healthy control subjects (Pollak et al. 1997; Satlin et al. 1991; Van Someren et al. 1996; Witting et al. 1990). In an-other study, the severity of sundowning in a group of patients with late-stage AD correlated with lower amplitudes of the locomotor circadian rhythm (Satlin et al. 1992). These objective findings are consistent with the clinical observations of an association between disturbed sleep and sun-downing in patients with dementia and consistent with a physiological basis for these abnormalities in the circadian timekeeping system.

The normal circadian organization of sleep is coupled to the circadian rhythm of core body temperature (Czeisler et al. 1980). Published studies of the temperature cycle in patients with AD are few in number, and their find-ings are not consistent with regard to amplitude and phase (Okawa et al. 1991; Prinz et al. 1984, 1992; Touitou et al. 1986). However, the lack of agree-ment in these reports may have been caused by the inclusion of patients with different degrees of dementia or of subgroups with different behav-ioral abnormalities. A study that found no overall difference in the ampli-tude of the core body-temperature circadian rhythm in 28 patients with AD compared with 10 control subjects identified a subgroup of AD patients with large mean time differences between the acrophases of their activity and temperature cycles (Satlin et al. 1995). This subgroup had lower tem-perature amplitudes and greater activity during the night. These findings suggest that a subgroup of patients with AD who have impaired circadian function may be at increased risk for sleep and behavioral disturbances by virtue of a desynchrony between the circadian cycles of temperature and ac-tivity. The basis of this desynchrony may lie in changes in the relative phase of the two rhythms, reductions of rhythm amplitude, or both.

Circadian abnormalities in patients with AD may have a neuropatho-logical correlate. Extensive experimental evidence suggests that the ana-tomic location of the circadian oscillator in mammalian species is in the suprachiasmatic nuclei (SCN) of the anterior hypothalamus (Moore 1982).

This pacemaker drives the circadian cycle of core body temperature, coordinates the synchrony of this rhythm with the sleep–wake cycle, and maintains its entrainment to the external environment (Czeisler et al. 1980). One neuropathologic study of the human SCN found a 60% decrease in nucleus volume and a 73% decrease in total SCN cell number in the brains of patients with AD compared with brains from matched healthy elderly control subjects (Swaab et al. 1985). Another study of the SCN found neurofibrillary tangles, the characteristic pathologic sign of AD (Stopa et al. 1989). Evidence from animal studies suggests that AD pathological changes can result in disruptions of circadian rhythmicity. Rats that received grafts into the SCN of genetically transformed cells that overexpress beta-amyloid had altered activity patterns, with abnormally high levels of activity during the light phase (normal sleeping time) and a disrupted circadian pattern (Tate et al. 1992).

From these findings, it may be hypothesized that sleep–wake cycle disruptions and sundowning in patients with AD may be caused by degeneration of circadian pacemaker function that leads to desynchrony of circadian rhythms. A central mechanism is suggested by the range of circadian rhythms affected in patients with AD, the changes in both amplitude and phase of these rhythms, and the degeneration of the anatomic pacemaker in the SCN. However, two other mechanisms are possible. First, disturbances in the synchrony of circadian rhythms may result from inadequate input to the SCN. The major external entraining stimulus for human circadian rhythms is bright light, which reaches the SCN through a direct tract from the retina through the optic nerve (Sadun et al. 1984). One group of investigators has found widespread axonal degeneration in the optic nerves of patients with AD (Hinton et al. 1986). There also is evidence that patients with AD are exposed to only about two-thirds the duration of bright light received by healthy younger subjects (Bliwise et al. 1993; Campbell et al. 1988) and that this deficiency is associated with less stable circadian rhythms (Van Someren et al. 1996). Second, altered circadian rhythms may result from dysfunction in the efferents from the SCN to its target organs or in those organs themselves. Most of the SCN efferents project to neighboring regions of the hypothalamus, but the mechanism through which these projections lead to the overt expression of circadian rhythmicity is as yet poorly worked out.

Rationale for Bright Light Therapy

The temporal nature of sundowning and its association with sleep disturbances and abnormal circadian rhythms suggest that treatments that strengthen the normal pacemaking function of the endogenous circadian oscillator may be beneficial in patients with this syndrome. One such treatment is bright light. Bright light exposure may theoretically reduce agitation and sleep disorders in patients with dementia by:

1. Providing a stronger external entraining signal to the circadian timekeeping mechanism to overcome either the age-associated loss of retinal input caused by degeneration of the optic nerve or the tendency of patients with dementia to be exposed to less environmental light.
2. Restoring to normal the reduced amplitude of the endogenous circadian oscillator associated with degeneration of the pacemaker cells in the SCN. Amplitude is believed to reflect the stability of a circadian rhythm. Properly timed bright light exposure may augment the amplitude of the circadian temperature rhythm (Czeisler et al. 1987). This effect is postulated to account for the antidepressant effects of phototherapy in SAD (Rosenthal et al. 1990) and the improvement with bright light in sleep maintenance insomnia (Campbell et al. 1993).
3. Phase shifting the endogenous oscillator to restore an appropriate relationship between the timing of the body temperature rhythm and an environmentally appropriate sleep–wake cycle. This effect is believed important in treating sleep disturbance in elderly patients (Campbell et al. 1993; Cooke et al. 1998).
4. Providing an activating effect during the day that results in more sustained alertness, less confusion and agitation, and more physical activity. Patients who sleep less during the day may sleep more soundly at night.
5. Preventing the age-related loss of vasopressin-expressing neurons in the SCN. This effect has recently been found in experiments with rats (Lucassen et al. 1995).

These theoretical considerations have led to the use of bright light therapy in several studies of patients with AD and multi-infarct dementia (MID) over the past few years. In general, these studies have focused on the alleviation of sleep disturbances, but agitation has also been measured. Techniques have included the use of light boxes, light visors, and increased overall room illumination. The intensity, duration, and timing of the light treatment have generally been those used in successful studies in patients with SAD (most often 2 hours of exposure to about 2,000 lux in either the early morning or evening). Patients have been studied in both institutional and community settings. So far, the results have been encouraging but equivocal.

A Review of Clinical Studies

A group of investigators in Japan conducted the most extensive studies. In one study, 14 inpatients with dementia (either multi-infarct or AD) who also met DSM-III-R (American Psychiatric Association 1987) criteria for insomnia disorder or sleep–wake schedule disorder and for whom medication treatment had failed were treated with 2 hours of morning bright light for 4 weeks and then followed up for an additional 2 weeks (Mishima et al. 1994). Nurses recorded sleep and behavior hourly throughout the 2-month period of the study. Serum melatonin levels were measured at midnight and noon before the light therapy and during the last week of light therapy. Behavior disorder mean scores declined from 23.9 to 11.6. Total sleep time and nocturnal sleep time increased and remained increased after the treatment was discontinued; daytime sleep time decreased during treatment but was no longer significantly decreased after the light therapy was stopped. There were no changes in melatonin levels with the light treatment. The association between the decreased frequency of behavioral disturbances and the improvement in sleep parameters, without a change in melatonin levels to indicate a change in the function of the endogenous circadian oscillator, suggests that the morning light increased daytime alertness and reduced daytime sleep, thereby causing a consolidation of sleep at night, with a consequent reduction in episodes of agitation.

Other studies by the same group included the measurement of oral temperature several times during the day. Although oral temperature may not reflect the functioning of the circadian pacemaker as accurately as core body temperature, these observations can provide useful preliminary data. In one study, eight inpatients with dementia (four with AD and four with multi-infarct dementa), irregular sleep–wake rhythms, and behavioral agitation had much greater variations in daily temperature (recorded orally at midnight, 4:00 A.M., 10:00 A.M., and 6:00 P.M.) than seven elderly patients without dementia (Okawa et al. 1989). After baseline measurements, patients were treated with social interaction therapy by the nurses, followed by phototherapy for those patients who did not respond. Treatment consisted of 2,000 lux every morning between 9:00 and 11:00 A.M. for 2–6 months. One patient with multi-infarct dementia responded to increased social contact, and the other three responded to light treatment; only one patient with AD responded to both social contact and phototherapy. There was corresponding improvement in the body temperature rhythm in only one patient with multi-infarct dementia whose sleep improved.

Another study compared the effects of morning (9:00–11:00 A.M.; 21 patients) or evening (5:00–7:00 P.M.; 6 patients) bright light (2,500 lux) in patients drawn from a group of 23 with moderate to severe dementia and 5 with slight or no dementia. All had sleep–wake cycle disturbances; the group with moderate or severe dementia had more marked oral temperature fluctuations (Hozumi et al. 1990). Morning light was reported to be effective in 11 of 21 patients, and evening light was not effective in any of the 6 patients treated. There were no changes in the rhythms of temperature or serum melatonin with treatment. Overall in these two studies the greater effectiveness of morning than evening light, the failure to find changes in temperature or melatonin cycles, and the similar effects of light and social interaction therapy are evidence that light therapy may have exerted its primary effect through a general increase in daytime activity and alertness, with the secondary effect of improved nighttime sleep.

Objective measurements of locomotor activity were used in a study of 10 residents with AD in an inpatient dementia unit (Satlin et al. 1992). All were identified by nursing staff as sundowners; most of the patients began pacing or yelling between 2:00 and 4:00 P.M. Patients also exhibited sleep disturbances characterized by frequent daytime napping and nighttime awakenings. Nurses performed daily ratings each shift (day, evening, and night) for agitation and sleep–wakefulness disturbances and also recorded all use of restraints and as-needed medication. Locomotor activity was recorded for 48 hours at the conclusion of a baseline week, the treatment week, and a posttreatment week. Treatment consisted of sitting in a geri-chair facing a light box that provided exposure to approximately 1,500–2,000 lux from 7:00 to 9:00 P.M. each evening for 7 days.

Clinical ratings of sleep wakefulness on the evening shift improved with light treatment in 8 of the 10 patients. There was a statistically significant decline in the overall mean score from baseline to the treatment week, with a further small decline during the posttreatment week. This finding was supported by some of the objective measures obtained from the activity monitor data. Intradaily variability decreased during the treatment week in 9 patients but returned to baseline during the posttreatment week. Interdaily stability did not change. The amplitude of the rest–activity cycle increased from baseline to the light treatment week in 7 patients, with a statistically significant change in the overall mean values. Clinical ratings of agitation, use of restraints, and use of as-needed medication did not change on any shift.

A composite baseline score for the severity of sundowning was calculated by subtracting the summed baseline daytime shift scores on all four clinical measures (sleep–wake pattern, agitation, use of restraints, and use of as-needed medication) from the summed baseline week evening shift scores. One patient had a neutral sundowning score (indicating no sundowning pattern); the scores of the other patients were all positive, indicating that behaviors were, in fact, worse in the evening. The severity of sundowning at baseline correlated with lower relative amplitudes of the rest–activity circadian cycle. A positive correlation also was found between the severity of sundowning at baseline and the degree of improvement during both the light treatment week and the posttreatment week.

This pilot study used an open-treatment, uncontrolled design. However, improvements in sleep–wake measures during the treatment week persisted into the posttreatment week, suggesting that the nurse ratings were not influenced by the presence of the light treatment itself. In addition, the nurses' clinical ratings were partially corroborated by the data from the activity monitor. The correlations between more severe sundowning at baseline and both reduced amplitude of the circadian rest–activity cycle and clinical improvement suggest that sundowning may be associated with disturbed circadian rhythms and that the severity of these disturbances may predict response to bright light. The effectiveness of evening light in this study suggests that the mechanism of improvement was probably not through homeostatic regulation of sleep. It is possible that the light exerted its effect by phase delaying the circadian core body temperature cycle, restoring a more normal phase relationship between this cycle and a phase-delayed rest–activity rhythm. Other possible mechanisms are an increase in the amplitude of the endogenous circadian oscillator or an entraining effect of the change in the daily routine.

To minimize the possibility of placebo effects associated with the administration of bright light therapy by seating patients in front of a light box, investigators in the Netherlands studied the effect of indirect whole-day unattended bright light. The light was administered by increasing the illumination in the living room of an inpatient psychogeriatric ward where patients spent most of their waking hours (Van Someren et al. 1997). A total of 22 patients with severe dementia (16 with AD, 3 with multi-infarct dementia, 2 with alcoholic dementia, and 1 with normal pressure hydrocephalus) were evaluated with actigraph recordings at baseline and at the end of the third week after installation of the increased lighting. They were then evaluated in the fourth week after replacement of the original lighting. No clinical assessments of either sleep or behavior were made. Light exposure was measured at one time point between 9:00 and 11:00 A.M. every day during the assessment periods, and a weekly average was calculated for each patient. Light intensity at eye level was found to be about 1,100 lux during the treatment week compared with roughly 400 lux during the baseline and posttreatment weeks.

The strongest overall predictor of response was the presence of a severe visual deficit, which was associated with a lack of effectiveness of the bright light. After excluding from further analyses the five patients who had such visual deficits, comparisons of the variable means during the light treatment week with those of the pooled baseline and posttreatment weeks found a significant increase in interdaily stability, a decrease in intradaily variability, and no change in the rest–activity rhythm amplitude. The results suggest that bright light provided a stronger entraining signal to the rest–activity rhythm than the usual lighting available on the inpatient unit. The failure to find a change in amplitude may have been caused by the timing of the light treatment, which was distributed throughout the day rather than administered as a pulse. Although these results are promising, they are also difficult to interpret in the absence of any clinical measures to suggest whether the objective findings of change were associated with improvement in sleep or behavior.

The studies described above included only institutionalized patients, raising the possibility that negative findings may have been caused by the patients' advanced stage of dementia. In a pilot study of five patients with AD residing in the community, circadian rest–activity rhythms were continuously monitored and bright light treatment was administered for 2 hours every morning (immediately on awakening) for 10 days using a Bio-brite Light Visor (Colenda et al. 1997). The investigators hypothesized that morning light would phase advance the circadian rhythm of rest–activity (which they assumed to be delayed in patients with AD) and that the alerting qualities of timed light exposure might enable these patients to stay awake during the day and therefore have more consolidated sleep at night. None of the five patients had changes from baseline in the number of nighttime awakenings or in the expected direction for acrophase, mesor, or amplitude of the circadian rest–activity rhythm. The authors hypothesized that their results may have been caused by improper timing of the light administration or an inadequate length of time for the light exposure. It is also possible that although the light visors were well tolerated, they might not have provided the expected amount of actual light delivery to the retina.

Patients in most of these studies were selected on the basis of baseline sleep disturbance. In a study that focused primarily on agitation, six patients with moderate to severe dementia were observed during a 3-day baseline period, 10 days of morning (9:30 to 11:30 A.M.) bright light treatment, and 5 days of posttreatment follow-up, followed by a repetition of this entire sequence (Lovell et al. 1995). Treatment was administered by a light box placed 1 meter from the patients. Behavior was rated 4 hours a day at 15-minute intervals from 4:00 to 8:00 P.M. Overall, agitation was significantly lower on light treatment days than on nontreatment days; in the first treatment period, four patients improved and two worsened. In the second treatment period, all six patients improved. Patients generally returned to their baseline levels of agitation by the second posttreatment day. Patients with more severe baseline agitation appeared more responsive to the treatment.

None of these studies reported any increase in agitation associated with the exposure to bright light. However, agitation and the development of hypomania have been noted in patients using light therapy for SAD (Labbate et al. 1994). Another important possible adverse effect of light treatment is acute ocular damage. This problem can be minimized by the use of lights that filter out the ultraviolet spectrum (Lee et al. 1997) and by avoiding the concomitant use of medications that are photosensitizing in ocular tissues, such as tricyclic and heterocyclic compounds (Reme et al. 1996) and melatonin (Leino et al. 1984). These precautions have direct clinical relevance because tricyclic compounds such as antipsychotics and antidepressants are commonly used for agitation in patients with dementia and melatonin has begun to receive attention as a possible hypnotic agent.

Conclusions

The results of the available studies of bright light in dementia patients with sundowning, sleep disturbance, or both may be interpreted to reach the following general conclusions:

- Preliminary and largely uncontrolled evidence suggests that bright light treatment may ameliorate agitation and sleep disorders in some patients with dementia.
- The clinical effect appears to be modest, but greater or more consistent effects may require individualized timing of the light treatment, selection of patient subgroups with underlying circadian pathology, and restriction of treatment to patients with intact visual systems.
- Studies so far have used light intensities, durations, and timing that are derived from successful studies in patients with SAD; nothing is known about whether different treatment parameters are needed in patients with dementia.
- Some evidence suggests that patients with multi-infarct dementia may respond better than patients with dementia and AD, but the data are too scant to confirm this hypothesis.

- Both morning and evening light have been found to be effective, and no evidence exists on which to base a selection of one or the other in individual patients.
- Bright light may improve symptoms either through an activating effect or by effects on the amplitude or phase of circadian rhythms. These circadian effects may be exerted at the level of input to the SCN or in the SCN itself, and they may involve mechanisms of rhythm entrainment or synchronization.
- Light visors, which may only be practical in patients with earlier-stage disease, have so far not been found effective. However, careful attention must be given to ensuring that an adequate amount of light reaches the retina when such devices are used. Overall increased room illumination appears to be a practical approach for use in institutional settings.
- No deleterious effect of bright light treatment in patients with dementia has been found in reported studies to date.

Summary Recommendations

Bright light therapy is a promising but as yet unproven treatment for the agitation and sleep disorders often found in patients with dementia. The available data are intriguing, but they cannot yet be translated into clear clinical recommendations. Future studies should make use of blinded raters and objective measures of outcome, and they need to define the correct timing, amount, and mode of administration of the light therapy.

Practicing clinicians should consider bright light therapy as an experimental procedure in patients with dementia. If such treatment is to be used, it should be done as part of a well-designed study with the aim of generating useful knowledge about the efficacy and safety of the procedure. Institutions that set up bright light therapy rooms should do so as part of a research program with the same aims. It is hoped that researchers, clinicians, nursing home administrators, and caregivers will find the information in this chapter to be a sound basis for evaluating future research in this area and for formulating clinical guidelines as they become supportable by data.

References

American Psychiatric Association: Diagnostic and Statistical Manual of Mental Disorders, 2nd Edition. Washington, DC, American Psychiatric Association, 1968

American Psychiatric Association: Diagnostic and Statistical Manual of Mental Disorders, 3rd Edition, Revised. Washington, DC, American Psychiatric Association, 1987

Ancoli-Israel S, Parker L, Sinaee R, et al: Sleep fragmentation in patients from a nursing home. J Gerontol 44:M18–M21, 1989

Bliwise DL, Carroll JS, Lee KA, et al: Sleep and "sundowning" in nursing home patients with dementia. Psychiatry Res 48:277–292, 1993

Cameron DE: Studies in senile nocturnal delirium. Psychiatr Q 15:47–53, 1941

Campbell SS, Kripke DF, Gillin JC, et al: Exposure to light in healthy elderly subjects and Alzheimer's patients. Physiol Behav 42:141–144, 1988

Campbell SS, Dawson D, Anderson MW: Alleviation of sleep maintenance insomnia with timed exposure to bright light. J Am Geriatr Soc 41:829–836, 1993

Cohen-Mansfield J, Marx MS: The relationship between sleep disturbances and agitation in a nursing home. Journal of Aging and Health 2:42–57, 1990

Cohen-Mansfield J, Watson V, Meade W, et al: Does sundowning occur in residents of an Alzheimer's unit? Int J Geriatr Psychiatry 4:293–298, 1989

Colenda CC, Cohen W, McCall WV, et al: Phototherapy for patients with Alzheimer disease with disturbed sleep patterns: results of a community-based pilot study. Alzheimer Dis Assoc Disord 11:175–178, 1997

Cooke KM, Kreydatus MA, Atherton A, et al: The effect of evening light exposure on the sleep of elderly women expressing sleep complaints. J Behav Med 21:103–114, 1998

Cornelissen G, Touitou Y, Tritsch G, et al: Circadian rhythms of adenosine deaminase activity in human erythrocytes: a transverse study on young, elderly and senile demented subjects. Ric Clin Lab 15:365–374, 1985

Czeisler CA, Weitzman ED, Moore-Ede MD, et al: Human sleep: its duration and organization depend on its circadian phase. Science 210:1264–1267, 1980

Czeisler CA, Kronauer RE, Mooney JJ, et al: Biologic rhythm disorders, depression and phototherapy: a new hypothesis. Psychiatr Clin North Am 10:687–709, 1987

Evans LK: Sundown syndrome in institutionalized elderly. J Am Geriatr Soc 35:101–108, 1987

Feinberg I, Koresko RL, Heller N: EEG sleep patterns as a function of normal and pathological aging in man. J Psychiatr Res 5:107–144, 1967

Hinton DR, Sadun AA, Blanks JC, et al: Optic nerve degeneration in Alzheimer's disease. N Engl J Med 315:485–487, 1986

Hozumi S, Okawa M, Mishima K, et al: Phototherapy for elderly patients with dementia and sleep-wake rhythm disorders: a comparison between morning and evening light exposure. Jpn J Psychiatry Neurol 44:813–814, 1990

Labbate LA, Lafer B, Thibault A, et al: Side effects induced by bright light treatment for seasonal affective disorder. J Clin Psychiatry 55:189–191, 1994

Lee TM, Chan CC, Paterson JG, et al: Spectral properties of phototherapy for seasonal affective disorder: a meta-analysis. Acta Psychiatr Scand 96:117–121, 1997

Leino M, Aho IM, Kari E, et al: Effects of melatonin and 6-methoxy-tetrahydro-beta-carboline in light induced retinal damage: a computerized morphometric method. Life Sci 35:1997–2001, 1984

Lewy AJ, Sack RL, Miller S, et al: Antidepressant and circadian phase-shifting effects of light. Science 235:352–354, 1987

Little JT, Satlin A, Sunderland T, et al: Sundown syndrome in severely demented patients with probable Alzheimer's disease. J Geriatr Psychiatry Neurol 8:103–106, 1995

Loewenstein RJ, Weingartner H, Gillin JC, et al: Disturbances of sleep and cognitive functioning in patients with dementia. Neurobiol Aging 3:371–377, 1982

Lovell BB, Ancoli-Israel S, Gevirtz R: Effect of bright light treatment on agitated behavior in institutionalized elderly subjects. Psychiatry Res 57:7–12, 1995

Lucassen PJ, Hofman MA, Swaab DF: Increased light intensity prevents the age related loss of vasopressin-expressing neurons in the rat suprachiasmatic nucleus. Brain Res 693:261–266, 1995

Mishima K, Okawa M, Hishikawa Y, et al: Morning bright light therapy for sleep and behavior disorders in elderly patients with dementia. Acta Psychiatr Scand 89:1–7, 1994

Moore RY: The suprachiasmatic nucleus and the organization of a circadian system. Trends Neurosci 5:404–407, 1982

Okawa M, Mishima K, Shimizu T, et al: Sleep-waking rhythm disorders and their phototherapy in elderly patients with dementia. Jpn J Psychiatry Neurol 43:293–295, 1989

Okawa M, Mishima K, Hishikawa Y, et al: Circadian rhythm disorders in sleep-waking and body temperature in elderly patients with dementia and their treatment. Sleep 14:478–485, 1991

Pollak CP, Stokes PE: Circadian rest-activity rhythms in demented and nondemented older community residents and their caregivers. J Am Geriatr Soc 45:446–452, 1997

Prinz PN, Peskind ER, Vitaliano PP, et al: Changes in the sleep and waking EEGs of nondemented and demented elderly subjects. J Am Geriatr Soc 30:86–93, 1982a

Prinz PN, Vitaliano PP, Vitiello MV, et al: Sleep, EEG and mental function changes in senile dementia of the Alzheimer's type. Neurobiol Aging 3:361–370, 1982b

Prinz PN, Christie C, Smallwood R, et al: Circadian temperature variation in healthy aged and in Alzheimer's disease. J Gerontol 39:30–35, 1984

Prinz PN, Moe KE, Vitiello MV, et al: Entrained body temperature rhythms are similar in mild Alzheimer's disease, geriatric onset depression and normal aging. J Geriatr Psychiatry Neurol 5:65–71, 1992

Rebok GW, Rovner BW, Folstein MF: Sleep disturbance and Alzheimer's disease: relationship to behavioral problems. Aging (Milano) 3:193–196, 1991

Reme CE, Rol P, Grothmann K, et al: Bright light therapy in focus: lamp emission spectra and ocular safety. Technol Health Care 4:403–413, 1996

Rosenthal NE, Levendosky AA, Skwerer J, et al: Effects of light treatment on core body temperature in seasonal affective disorder. Biol Psychiatry 27:39–50, 1990

Sadun AA, Schaechter JD, Smith TH: A retinohypothalamic pathway in man: light mediation of circadian rhythms. Brain Res 302:371–377, 1984

Satlin A, Teicher MH, Lieberman HR, et al: Circadian locomotor activity rhythms in Alzheimer's disease. Neuropsychopharmacology 5:115–126, 1991

Satlin A, Volicer L, Ross V, et al: Bright light treatment of behavioral and sleep disturbances in patients with Alzheimer's disease. Am J Psychiatry 149:1028–1032, 1992

Satlin A, Volicer L, Stopa EG, et al: Circadian locomotor activity and core-body temperature rhythms in Alzheimer's disease. Neurobiol Aging 16:765–771, 1995

Souetre E, Salvati E, Belugou J-L, et al: Circadian rhythms in depression and recovery: evidence for blunted amplitude as the main chronobiological abnormality. Psychiatry Res 28:263–278, 1989

Stopa EG, Tate-Ostroff B, Walcott EC, et al: Human suprachiasmatic nuclei in Alzheimer's disease. J Neuropathol Exp Neurol 48:327, 1989

Swaab DF, Fliers E, Partiman TS: The suprachiasmatic nucleus of the human brain in relation to sex, age and senile dementia. Brain Res 342:37–44, 1985

Tate B, Aboody-Guterman KS, Morris AM, et al: Disruption of circadian regulation by brain grafts that overexpress Alzheimer B/A4 amyloid. Proc Natl Acad Sci USA 89:7090–7094, 1992

Touitou Y, Sulon J, Bogdan A, et al: Adrenal circadian system in young and elderly human subjects: a comparative study. J Endocrinol 93:201–210, 1982

Touitou Y, Reinberg A, Bogdan A, et al: Age-related changes in both circadian and seasonal rhythms of rectal temperature, wth special reference to senile dementia of Alzheimer type. Gerontology 32:110–118, 1986

Van Someren EJW, Hagebeuk EEO, Lijzenga C, et al: Circadian rest-activity rhythm disturbances in Alzheimer's disease. Biol Psychiatry 40:259–270, 1996

Van Someren EJW, Kessler A, Mirmiran M, et al: Indirect bright light improves circadian rest-activity rhythm disturbances in demented patients. Biol Psychiatry 41:955–963, 1997

Vitiello MV, Prinz PN, Williams DE, et al: Sleep disturbances in patients with mild-stage Alzheimer's disease. J Gerontol 45:M131–M138, 1990

Vitiello MV, Bliwise DL, Prinz PN: Sleep in Alzheimer's disease and the sundown syndrome. Neurology 42(suppl 6):83–94, 1992

Witting W, Kwa IH, Eikelenboom P, et al: Alterations in the circadian rest-activity rhythm in aging and Alzheimer's disease. Biol Psychiatry 27:563–572, 1990

CHAPTER 10

Serotonergic Agents

Kari L. Franson, Pharm.D.
Deanna Chesley, Pharm.D.
John S. Kennedy, M.D., F.R.C.P.C.

In this chapter we review the rationale behind using serotonergic agents for mild behavioral disturbances in patients with Alzheimer's disease (AD) by discussing the pathophysiology, pharmacology, and clinical data regarding these drugs.

The pathological process that produces AD is complex and is noted to result in significant neurotransmitter losses (acetylcholine is down approximately 90%; serotonin, 50%–70%; norepinephrine, 30%–70%; and γ-amino-butyric acid [GABA], 50%). Although serotonin is not the most profoundly affected neurotransmitter, there is abundant evidence for central serotonin depletion in patients with AD. There are 1) substantial neuronal losses in the raphe nuclei; 2) reduced central nervous system (CNS) concentrations of 5-hydroxytryptamine (5-HT) and its 5-hydroxyindoleacetic acid (5-HIAA) metabolite, especially in the temporal cortex (Arora et al. 1991; Cross 1990); and 3) reduced H-ketanserine-labeled 5-HT$_2$ receptor levels (a relatively early change in the course of the disease), although receptor affinity remains unchanged (Cross 1990). Conversely, the number of 5-HT uptake sites on blood platelets is significantly increased in patients with mild and moderate dementia of the Alzheimer type (DAT) compared with normal control subjects (Arora et al. 1991). This serotonergic depletion has been found to be associated with aggressive behaviors.

Palmer et al. (1988) found evidence of lower levels of 5-HT in the brains of aggressive patients with AD in comparison with nonaggressive patients. Thus, drugs that increase the central serotonin neurotransmission would theoretically be of benefit. Serotonin abnormalities are associated with panic, anxiety, impulsivity, and aggressiveness characteristic of various psychiatric conditions (van Pragg et al. 1990). Patients with these conditions have responded to agents that increase serotonin neurotransmission, inhibit 5-HT_2 receptors, or stimulate the 5-HT_{1A} receptors. These pharmacological effects can be achieved with the serotonin selective reuptake inhibitor (SSRI) antidepressants and trazodone, nefazodone, and buspirone. Eichelman's (1987) review of the literature also stated that by increasing tryptophan (a serotonin precursor), lithium could also modulate aggression.

Antidepressants

Trazodone

Trazodone is a phenylpiperazine agent with complex serotonergic actions. The drug is a weak serotonin 5-HT reuptake inhibitor compared with SSRIs such as fluoxetine. It also is thought to exhibit 5HT_2 receptor antagonism and, via its metabolite M-chlorophenylpiperazine, $5\text{-HT}_{2A/2C}$ receptor agonism. The consequences of blocking the 5-HT_2 receptor include decreased agitation, anxiety, panic attacks, and insomnia (Stahl 1998). Trazodone also causes sedation, which may contribute to its antiagitation mechanism of action. This effect may be mediated by central blockade of alpha-1, histamine, or 5-HT_2 receptors. Finally, trazodone may decrease agitation behavior through its antidepressant effect.

Literature Review

Numerous case reports and open studies have shown trazodone to be effective in the treatment of agitation (Table 10–1). Unfortunately, no published placebo-controlled, double-blind trials currently exist. The dosages reported ranged from 150 to 500 mg/day and as low as 75 mg/day in three or four divided doses. Side effects occurred rarely, with sedation and orthostasis reported most commonly. The time until clinical effect appeared to be approximately 2–4 weeks.

    Pinner and Rich (1988) evaluated the effects of trazodone on aggressive behavior in seven inpatients (mean age, 63 years) with organic mental disorders. Three of the seven patients demonstrated a positive clinical response as determined through review of clinical records. Dosages were titrated to response and appearance of side effects and ranged from 250 to 300 mg/day. Duration of therapy until maximum improvement ranged

Table 10-1. Treatment of agitation with trazodone

Study	Dosage, mg/day[a]	Diagnosis (number of subjects)	Behavior	Benefit
Simpson and Foster (1986)	200, 400	DAT (2)	Combativeness, shouting, agitation	Improvement in all symptoms
Tingle (1986)	300	Pick's disease (1)	Hostility, withdrawal, delusions	Improvement in all symptoms
Greenwald et al. (1986)	300	Moderately advanced dementia (1)	Dysphoria, screaming, hitting themselves in the head, echolalia	Improvement in all symptoms
Pinner and Rich (1988)	200–400	Mixed OBS (3), schizophrenia (1), alcoholic dementia (2)	Physical aggression	Decreased aggression in three subjects
Lebert et al. (1994)	75	DAT (13)	Irritability, anxiety, restlessness, affective disturbance	Improvement in all symptoms
Houlihan et al. (1994)	Mean = 172	PDD (13), MID (3), dementia (6)	Irritability, aggression, restlessness, vocalization, sleep problems, wandering	Improvement in behavioral symptoms

Note.   DAT=dementia of Alzheimer's type; MID=multi-infarct dementia; OBS=organic brain syndrome; PDD= primary degenerative dementia.
[a]Three to four times per day.
Source.   Adapted from Tariot 1996.

from 30 to 43 days. The four remaining patients either did not respond to trazodone or had an undetermined response. No side effects occurred that could be definitely attributed to the drug, and the dose in the nonresponders was not increased further because of side effects. The authors concluded that trazodone should be used with caution in patients with aggression, because no discernible characteristic could be identified for responders versus nonresponders. The authors also concluded that further controlled trials are needed.

Lebert et al. (1994) treated 13 patients (mean age, 70 years) with presumptive DAT and affective and behavioral disturbance with 25 mg of trazodone three times daily for 10 weeks. Behavioral and affective disturbance was evaluated at baseline and after 10 weeks of drug therapy via interview with the patient and caregiver using the Gottfries-Brane-Steen and the Jouvent's Depressed Mood scales. Side effects were also assessed after 10 weeks of trazodone therapy. There was a significant reduction in postdrug effects, including, most notably, emotional lability, irritability, anxiety, and restlessness. No side effects were noted that could be attributed to the drug. The authors concluded that trazodone appeared to be effective in decreasing both emotional and behavioral disturbances, but further controlled trials were needed.

Dosage

Traditionally, trazodone has been used in the treatment of depression in doses of 150–400 mg/day and as a hypnotic in doses of 50–100 mg before bedtime (Gelman et al. 1997; Schatzberg and Nemeroff 1995). Primary literature has reported the use of trazodone for treatment of agitation in doses of 75–500 mg/day in three or four divided doses.

Side Effects

Trazodone does not interact with muscarinic receptors and therefore is devoid of anticholinergic side effects (Gelman et al. 1997; Schatzberg and Nemeroff 1995). Sedation is a relatively predictable side effect that may also be considered a therapeutic effect, depending on its degree and the functioning of the patient. Trazodone blocks alpha-1 adrenergic receptors, causing orthostasis and, potentially, dry mouth. Orthostasis is a particularly important side effect because it increases the risk of falls and bone fractures. Other cardiovascular side effects that may rarely occur in patients with preexisting cardiac disease are cardiac arrhythmias (isolated premature ventricular contractions, ventricular couplets, and short episodes of ventricular tachycardia). Therefore, caution is warranted when administering the drug in this patient population (Gelman et al. 1997). Lastly, trazodone may rarely cause priapism, with a prevalence of one in 6,000 patients. The greatest risk for priapism appears to be during initiation of therapy at low doses (<150 mg/day) (Schatzberg and Nemeroff 1995).

Significant Drug–Drug Interactions

Other CNS depressants may potentiate the sedative effect of trazodone (Gelman et al. 1997; Schatzberg and Nemeroff 1995). If the patient is taking a number of medications that cause sedation, it should be recognized that the dose of trazodone may need to be increased more slowly and cautiously. Because trazodone increases serotonin actions, it has the potential to cause serotonin syndrome when combined with buspirone, lithium, meperidine, and monoamine oxidase inhibitors. If these medications are used together, close monitoring is warranted. Additionally, although trazodone can cause orthostasis, it can also inhibit the antihypertensive action of clonidine (Gelman et al. 1997; Schatzberg and Nemeroff 1995). This combination is best avoided because of the variety of antihypertensives available to use as appropriate alternatives.

Nefazodone

Nefazodone is another phenylpiperazine agent with serotonergic effects similar to those of trazodone (Davis 1997; Stahl 1998). Nefazodone's side effect profile is also similar to trazodone's, except that nefazodone has less sedative properties than trazodone and less potential to cause both orthostasis and priapism. Nefazodone's more desirable side effect profile may be related to its effect of norephinephrine reuptake inhibition, which may counteract the effect of alpha-1 blockade and related side effects (Stahl 1998). Similar to trazodone, nefazodone has antianxiety and antidepressant actions. No case reports or studies directly assessing the effect of nefazodone in the treatment of patients with agitation could be identified. However, there is evidence of its efficacy in the treatment of anxiety and agitation symptoms associated with major depression (Fawcett 1995). Caution is warranted if nefazodone is used with benzodiazepines because nefazadone inhibits the cytochrome P450 3A4 isoenzyme. There is the potential for an increase in the level and therefore an increase in the effect of the benzodiazepine (Michalets 1998). Astemizole and cisapride are also drugs metabolized by the 3A4 isoenzyme group. Neither drug should be coadministered with nefazodone because of the risk of increased blood levels of the drugs, potentially leading to cardiac arrhythmias. Nefazodone also now has a black box warning about potential liver damage.

Selective Serotonin Reuptake Inhibitors

Murray and Raskind (1998) suggested that certain SSRIs (i.e., citalopram and fluvoxamine) may be effective for at least some noncognitive behavioral problems in patients with AD. Citalopram has been shown to block the reuptake of 5-HT into serotonergic neurons, with little effect on the uptake of norepinephrine or dopamine (Hyttel 1982). Presumed to be linked to its inhibition of CNS neuronal uptake of serotonin in vitro, citalopram has no significant affinity for adrenergic (alpha1, alpha2, beta) cholinergic, GABA, dopaminergic, histaminergic, serotonergic ($5\text{-}HT_{1A}$, $5\text{-}HT_{1B}$, $5\text{-}HT_2$), or benzodiazepine receptors. It also does not inhibit monoamine oxidase.

Literature Review

There are some preliminary reports of the clinical effects of drugs inhibiting neuronal 5-HT reuptake in patients with dementia. In an open, 2-week pilot study of a serotonin reuptake blocker without anticholinergic activity, 200 mg of alaproclate was given twice daily to 12 inpatients with AD whose behavioral problems were not specified. Five patients were judged to have improved, showing reduced irritability, reduced aggressiveness, and better tolerance to stress. Three patients dropped out (Bergman et al. 1983). However, a subsequent placebo-controlled, 4-week, parallel group, double-blind study of alaproclate given at the same dosage to 40 nursing home patients with either AD or multi-infarct dementia showed no efficacy for the drug (Dehlin et al. 1985).

In a multicenter Scandinavian study (Nyth and Gottfries 1990), the clinical efficacy of citalopram was investigated in 98 patients with moderate AD or DAT or vascular dementia using a placebo-controlled, parallel-group study. Patients with AD or DAT showed significant improvements in emotional blunting, confusion, irritability, anxiety, fear or panic, depressed mood, and restlessness after 4 weeks of treatment with citalopram. No significant effects of citalopram were noted in patients with vascular dementia. This was the first controlled study reporting that a selective 5-HT reuptake inhibitor seemed to have a beneficial effect in patients with dementia disorders.

In another Scandinavian study (Olafsson et al. 1992), the efficacy of fluvoxamine on cognitive functioning and behavioral changes was evaluated in a double-blind, placebo-controlled study of 46 patients with dementia. Fluvoxamine tended to be more effective than placebo on the target symptoms of confusion, irritability, anxiety, fear or panic, mood level, and restlessness. The differences between fluvoxamine and placebo, however, failed to reach the standard level of statistical significance. For both of the SSRIs described in these studies, citalopram and fluvoxamine, reduction in aggressiveness usually occurred quickly and without delay, suggesting that serotonin activation results in a direct effect on irritability and aggressiveness (Karlsson 1996). Despite the widespread use of the SSRIs, there is very little published empirical evidence for their effectiveness except regarding the use of citalopram and fluvoxamine for treating behavioral disturbances in elderly patients with dementia (Schneider and Sobin 1992).

Coccaro (1990) assessed the efficacy of open-label fluoxetine in the treatment of impulsive aggressive behavior in three patients with DSM-III-R (American Psychiatric Association 1987) criteria for personality disorder. These data suggested that fluoxetine may be a useful agent for the treatment of impulsive aggressive behavior. Swartz et al. (1997) studied the treatment of frontotemporal dementia with SSRIs. Eleven subjects meeting the Lund-Manchester clinical neuropsychological and neuroimaging criteria for frontotemporal dementia were treated with fluoxetine, sertraline, or paroxetine. After treatment, improvement was shown in disinhibition, depressive symptoms, carbohydrate craving, and compulsions in at least half of the subjects in which they had been present. The authors concluded that the behavioral symptoms of frontotemporal dementia may improve after treatment with SSRIs. However, one subject stopped sertraline treatment because of diarrhea, and another stopped paroxetine treatment because of increased anxiety. The presence of individual behavioral symptoms and the response of each symptom to SSRIs were unrelated to cognitive impairment as measured by baseline Mini-Mental State Examination score. Several studies suggest that SSRIs may be helpful in the management of noncognitive problem behaviors in elderly persons with AD.

Doses

In the previously mentioned dementia behavior studies, the dosing of the SSRIs did not differ from antidepressant dosing. Dosing was started lower to allow the clinicians to "start low and go slow." Clinical use suggests that citalopram can be started at 10 mg and increased to doses of 40 mg. Maximum dosages of citalopram are 80 mg/day. Fluvoxamine is used clinically at dosages between 50 and 300 mg/day. This dosage is split into two daily doses (Gelman et al. 1997; Schatzberg and Nemeroff 1995).

Side Effects

The SSRIs are all structurally unique and have diverse adverse-effect profiles. They commonly cause nausea, but this effect is normally self-limiting and can be minimized with a slow titration schedule. Fluvoxamine was found to cause somnolence, insomnia, nervousness, tremor, anorexia, vomiting, abnormal ejaculation, asthenia, and sweating. In studies of adults receiving citalopram, side effects included dry mouth, sleepiness, increase in sweating, and sexual problems in men. Not all SSRI agents are used to treat agitation in elderly individuals. Paroxetine is often avoided because of its high affinity for blocking muscarinic receptors. Clinicians use fluoxetine because it has a long half-life. Fluoxetine may accumulate in elderly patients. Sertraline has a favorable side effect profile in elderly patients; however, there is a paucity of data regarding its use in patients with dementia.

Significant Drug–Drug Interactions

Pharmaceutical manufacturing companies have well characterized the drug interactions with the SSRIs. Fluvoxamine interacts with medications that are eliminated by the CYP 1A2 isoenzyme, which includes theophylline, caffeine, and tacrine. CYP isoenzyme interactions with citalopram have not been found to be clinically significant.

Antianxiety Agents

Buspirone

Buspirone is an arylpiperazine derivative that has been traditionally used for the treatment of anxiety. Unlike benzodiazepines, buspirone does not appear to exhibit its mechanism of action via GABA but rather through the serotonin receptors and dopamine 2 (D_2) receptors. Its serotonergic effects are not fully understood, but they are currently best characterized as a partial agonism or mixed agonism and antagonism at the serotonin 1 receptor. The serotonergic actions may help to explain its potential role in the treatment of both agitation and depression. Buspirone's dopaminergic effects are also not fully understood, but they appear to be mixed D_2-receptor agonism and antagonism.

Literature Review

A few case reports and small studies have assessed the use of buspirone for the treatment of patients with agitation with favorable results. None were double-blind, placebo-controlled trials (Table 10–2).

Herrmann and Eryavec (1993) administered buspirone to 16 patients whose agitation symptoms had not responded to previous therapy. The patients' mean age was 78 years, their primary diagnosis was dementia,

Table 10–2. Buspirone for the treatment of agitation

Study (n)	Mean daily dose, mg	Time to maximum benefit	Outcome	Side effects
Cantillon et al. 1996 (28)	15	Not reported	Decrease in Anxiety Status Inventory, (buspirone) 11.1 vs. (haloperidol) 2.1; and in Brief Psychiatric Rating Scale tension subscale, (buspirone) 10.9 vs. (haloperidol) 1.6	Not reported
Herrmann and Eryavec 1993 (16)	27	Not reported	Improvement in Clinical Global Impression scale in 6 of 16 patients	Increased agitation (possible) Acute dystonia (possible)
Sakauye et al. 1993 (10)	30–40	5–7 weeks	22% decrease in Cohen-Mansfield Agitated Behavior Scale score	Nausea

and all had severe behavioral symptoms. Buspirone dose was initiated at 5 mg three times a day and titrated upward in response to clinical outcome, with minimum duration of therapy set at 1 month. The primary outcome was measured by the Clinical Global Impression Scale. Six patients were rated as very much or much improved in terms of decreased agitation and aggression. The remaining patients either did not respond or worsened. There were only two side effects that could be attributed, possibly, to buspirone: an acute dystonic reaction and paradoxical increased agitation. The average dosage of buspirone for all 16 patients was 27 mg/day.

Sakauye et al. (1993) studied the effects of buspirone for the treatment of agitation in 10 patients with dementia, mean age 82.7 years. The length of treatment was 12 weeks. Buspirone was initiated at 5 mg three times a day with weekly increases of 5 mg/day. The primary outcome was assessed at baseline and at the end of the study. It consisted of a rating on the Cohen-Mansfield Agitated Behavior Scale (C-MADS; Cohen-Mansfield and Billig 1986), a seven-point Likert scale for 13 behavioral factors. There was a 22% reduction in C-MADS scores from baseline to end of the study, which was statistically significant. The dose that demonstrated the maximum benefit was 30–40 mg/day, and the time to maximum benefit occurred by the fifth to seventh week. Nausea was the only reported side effect. The authors pointed out that a positive response to buspirone was highly variable between patients.

Cantillon et al. (1996) conducted a double-blind pilot study of buspirone versus haloperidol therapy for the treatment of agitation associated with DAT. A total of 28 nursing home residents were selected on the basis of high levels of psychomotor activity and intrusive physical and verbal aggression, which were classified as agitation. The mean age was 78 years, and the length of therapy with either study drug was 10 weeks. After a 1-week washout phase, the patients were randomly assigned to receive therapy with haloperidol 1.5 mg/day or buspirone 15 mg/day, with the possibility of dosage increase in the first 2 weeks based on clinical response. Outcome evaluations included scores on the Brief Psychiatric Rating Scale (BPRS) tension subscale and nurses' observations, which were recorded every 2 weeks. The mean dosages of buspirone and haloperidol were 15 mg/day and 1.3 mg/day, respectively. There were statistically greater decreases in the outcome scores on the tension subscale of the BPRS in favor of buspirone versus haloperidol. However, there were no significant differences in the changes associated with the nurses' observations or total BPRS scales between treatment groups, and no side effect occurred that could be attributed to either of the study drugs.

Although evidence indicates that buspirone may be effective in the treatment of patients with agitation, a well-constructed, large trial is needed to fully demonstrate efficacy. Also, there appears to be variation in response to buspirone, with some patients actually at risk of developing more agitation.

Doses

Buspirone is usually started at a subtherapeutic dose and titrated to its maintenance dose to prevent side effects. Usual starting doses are 10–15 mg/day in divided doses, and maintenance doses are 15–60 mg/day in two to three divided doses. Onset to therapeutic action is at about 4 weeks but may take up until 6 weeks on therapeutic doses. Studies assessing the effect of buspirone on agitation used doses of 15–40 mg/day.

Side Effects

The most commonly reported side effects are dizziness, drowsiness, headache, and nausea. Buspirone has been associated with a "syndrome of restlessness," which emphasizes the importance of monitoring for therapeutic improvement versus worsening (Gelman et al 1997).

Significant Drug–Drug Interactions

Buspirone should not be used in combination with monoamine oxidase inhibitors. Other centrally acting agents should be used with caution when combined with buspirone because such combinations have not yet been fully studied (Gelman et al 1997).

Conclusions

Few clinical trials have studied the use of serotonergic agents for behavioral disturbances in patients with dementia. Reasons for their efficacy are currently speculative. However, some data do demonstrate positive outcomes in patients who have received these agents. Antidepressant agents are worth trying, particularly in patients who present with depressive symptoms. Buspirone may be helpful in treating those with predominant anxiety symptoms. The potential benefits would probably outweigh the risks of side effects of these relatively safe agents. However, there is a significant risk associated with the high cost of therapy that does not improve the patients' state of well-being.

References

American Psychiatric Association: Diagnostic and Statistical Manual of Mental Disorder, 3rd Edition, Revised. Washington, DC, American Psychiatric Association, 1987

Arora RC, Emery OB, Meltzer HY: Serotonin uptake in the blood platelets of Alzheimer's disease patients. Neurology 41:1307–1309, 1991

Bergman I, Brane G, Gottfries CG, et al: A pharmacokinetic and biochemical study in patients with dementia of Alzheimer type. Psychopharmacology (Berlin) 80:279–283, 1983

Cantillon M, Brunswick R, Molina D, et al: Am J Geriatr Psychiatry 4:263–267, 1996

Coccaro EF: Fluoxetine treatment of impulsive aggression in DSM-III-R personality disorder patients (letter). J Clin Psychopharmacol 10:373–375, 1990

Cohen-Mansfield J, Billig N: Agitated behaviors in the elderly, I: a conceptual review. J Am Geriatr Soc 34:722–727, 1986

Cross AJ: Serotonin in Alzheimer-type dementia and other dementing illnesses. Ann N Y Acad Sci 600P:405–415, 1990

Davis R, Whittington R, Harriet B: Nefazodone. Drugs 53:608–636, 1997

Dehlin O, Hedenrud B, Jansson P, et al: A double-blind comparison of alaproclate and placebo in the treatment of patients with senile dementia. Acta Psychiatr Scand 71:190–196, 1985

Eichelman B: Neurochemical basis of aggressive behavior. Psychiatr Ann 17:371–374, 1987

Fawcett J, Marcus R, Anton S, et al: Response of anxiety and agitation symptoms during nefazodone treatment of major depression. J Clin Psychiatry 56(suppl 6):37–42, 1995

Gelman CR, Rumack BH, Hutchison TA (eds): DRUGDEX System. Englewood, CO, Micromedex, Inc., 1997

Greenwald B, Marin D, Silverman S: Serotonergic treatment of screaming and banging in dementia. Lancet 2:1464–1465, 1986

Herrmann N, Eryavec G: Buspirone in the management of agitation and aggression associated with dementia. Am J Geriatr Psychiatry 1:249–252, 1993

Houlihan D, Mulsant B, Sweet R, et al: A naturalistic study of trazodone in the treatment of behavioral complications of dementia. Am J Geriatr Psychiatry 2:74–85, 1994

Hyttel J: Citalopram: pharmacological profile of a specific serotonin uptake inhibitor with antidepressant activity. Prog Neuropsychopharmacol Biol Psychiatry 6:277–295, 1982

Karlsson I: Pharmacologic treatment of noncognitive symptoms of dementia. Acta Neurol Scand 165(suppl):101–104, 1996

Lebert F, Pasquier F, Petit H: Behavioral effects of trazodone in Alzheimer's disease. J Clin Psychiatry 55:536–538, 1994

Michalets E: Update: clinically significant cytochrome P-450 drug interactions. Pharmacotherapy 18:84–112, 1998

Murray A, Raskind: Psychopharmacology of noncognitive abnormal behaviors in Alzheimer's disease. J Clin Psychiatry 59(suppl 9):28–32, 1998

Nyth AL, Gottfries CG: The clinical efficacy of citalopram in treatment of emotional disturbances in dementia disorders. Br J Psychiatry 157:894–901, 1990

Olafsson K, Jorgensen S, Jensen HV, et al: Fluvoxamine in the treatment of demented elderly patients: a double-blind, placebo-controlled study. Acta Psychiatr Scand 85:453–456, 1992

Palmer AM, Stratman GC, Procter AW, et al: Possible neurotransmitter basis of behavioral changes in Alzheimer disease. Ann Neurol 23:616–620, 1988

Pinner E, Rich C: Effects of trazodone on aggressive behavior in seven patients with organic mental disorders. Am J Psychiatry 145:1295–1296, 1988

Sakauye K, Camp C, Ford P: Effects of buspirone on agitation associated with dementia. Am J Geriatr Psychiatry 1:82–84, 1993

Schatzberg AF, Nemeroff CB (eds): American Psychiatric Press Textbook of Psychopharmacology. Washington, DC, American Psychiatric Press, 1995

Schneider LS, Sobin PB: Non-neuroleptic treatment of behavioral symptoms and agitation in Alzheimer's disease and other dementias. Psychopharmacol Bull 28:71–79, 1992

Simpson D, Foster D: Improvement in organically disturbed behavior with trazodone treatment. J Clin Psychiatry 47:191–193, 1986

Stahl S: Psychopharmacology of Antidepressants. Gillingham, United Kingdom, Scribe Design, 1998

Swartz JR, Miller BL, Lesser IM, et al: Frontotemporal dementia: treatment response to serotonin selective reuptake inhibitors. J Clin Psychiatry 58:212–216, 1997

Tariot P: Treatment strategies for agitation and psychosis in dementia. J Clin Psychiatry 57(suppl):21–29, 1996

Tingle D: Trazodone in dementia (letter). J Clin Psychiatry 47:482, 1986

van Pragg HM, Asnis GM, Kahn RS, et al: Monoamines and abnormal behavior: a multi-aminergic perspective. Br J Psychiatry 157:723–734, 1990

CHAPTER 11

Mood Stabilizers

Steven P. Wengel, M.D.
David G. Folks, M.D.

Mood stabilizers are a recent addition to the armamentarium for agitation in dementia. Much of the existing literature about mood stabilizers for agitation consists of small case series or open trials. Additionally, some information is extrapolated from reports of use of these agents in younger individuals with traumatic brain injuries and associated aggressive or agitated behaviors.

Clinicians have observed parallels between the behavior seen in patients with dementia and the behavior that occurs in cognitively intact patients with bipolar disorder. In particular, both patient populations demonstrate psychomotor agitation, sleep disturbances, and abnormalities of speech. In those with agitated dementia, the speech abnormalities frequently take the form of purposeless, repetitive vocalizations rather than rapid speech or flight of ideas, but the common element is the loud and disruptive pattern of speech. These similarities have resulted in speculation that agitation in dementia may, in fact, be a form of "organic mania." The natural consequence of such a hypothesis is to treat patients with dementia-associated agitation with medications known to treat idiopathic mania.

Another rationale for mood stabilizers in the treatment of agitation is the role lithium, carbamazepine, valproate, and other agents play in facilitating GABAergic transmission (Janicak et al.1993). γ-Aminobutyric acid (GABA) is a major inhibitory neurotransmitter, so enhancing it is believed to have an ameliorating effect on agitation.

Lithium

Lithium has been reported to decrease agitation in a variety of conditions that involve cognitive impairment, including mental retardation, Korsakoff's syndrome, and impulsive behaviors in prison populations (Keltner and Folks 1997). Although well established as mood stabilizer, lithium has had limited use in treating agitation in patients with dementia. In their review, Schneider and Sobin (1991) noted that only 4 of 22 patients with Alzheimer's disease responded to lithium. One case involved an 87-year-old woman who improved rapidly with a serum lithium level of only 0.2 mEq/L. No controlled study has shown that lithium is effective in treating aggression. Lithium may be useful in treating aggression and irritability related to manic excitement. Its antiagitation and antiaggression effects are likely achieved at serum levels comparable with those used in treating bipolar disorder (i.e., 0.4 to 1.2 mEq/L). Lithium's antiagitation and antiaggression effects may augment the effects of other agents, including antidepressants, antipsychotics, or carbamazepine. Overall, there is little enthusiasm among researchers for pursuing larger controlled trials of lithium in patients with dementia because of lithium's limited efficacy and the significant risk of side effects in geriatric populations.

Side Effects

General Side Effects

Lithium as a treatment for agitation poses certain limitations with respect to side effects that may be prohibitive in many geriatric patients. Because lithium is a simple ion whose entry into the body is governed by the same physiological mechanisms as sodium, lithium reaches virtually all body tissues. Toxicity almost always occurs above levels of 2.0 mEq/L and may be seen even at "therapeutic" blood levels. Common side effects include nausea, dry mouth, diarrhea, and thirst. At higher therapeutic or toxic levels ataxia, confusion, myoclonus, and extrapyramidal symptoms (EPS) may emerge. Drowsiness, mild hand tremor, polyuria, weight gain and a bloated feeling, sleeplessness, and headaches are other relatively common side effects. A lithium tremor tends to be irregular in rhythm and amplitude and affects the fingers; jerky motions of the flexion and extension of fingers are also commonly associated. Side effects unrelated to serum levels include weight gain, a metallic taste in the mouth, edema of the hands and ankles, and pruritis. During lithium treatment, patients with edema of the ankles or lower legs generally have normal renal, cardiovascular, and hepatic function. This edema may appear spontaneously and may respond favorably to 25–50 mg twice daily of spironolactone, a specific aldosterone inhibitor that may attempt to normalize tubular reabsorption of sodium, which has some role in the formation of edema (Keltner and Folks 1997).

Cardiovascular Side Effects

Lithium produces flattening or inversion of T waves, which is usually benign. It can also slow conduction at the sinoatrial node and exacerbate underlying sick sinus syndrome. This effect may be enhanced in patients taking other medications (i.e., quinidine and digoxin) that alter sinus node conduction (Lenox and Manji 1995). Lithium may also exacerbate underlying ventricular irritability and potentially produce ventricular tachyarrythmias (Liptzin 1992).

Endocrine Side Effects

Lithium may be associated with the development of euthyroid goiter, hyperthyroidism with or without thyroid gland enlargement, or hypothyroidism. Thus, baseline measurements of thyroid function should be obtained. Hyperparathyroidism occurs less commonly; it has been reported in 20 cases (Lenox and Manji 1995).

Central Nervous System Side Effects

Elderly individuals appear to be at greater risk than younger persons for neurological side effects of lithium. Severe EPS such as muscle rigidity, flexed posture, and bradykinesia have been reported in elderly bipolar patients receiving lithium in the therapeutic range (Arya 1996; Holroyd and Smith 1995). These symptoms improved greatly within 5 days of stopping lithium. In another case, a 67-year-old man with bipolar disorder developed symptoms of Creutzfeldt-Jakob syndrome (i.e., progressive dementia, myoclonic jerks, and parkinsonism) while taking lithium. An electrocardiogram revealed generalized sharp waves that, along with the clinical features noted previously, reverted to normal when lithium was discontinued (Casanova et al. 1996).

Renal Side Effects

Renal insufficiency lengthens the half-life of lithium, necessitating reductions in dosage. Absorption and excretion of lithium are closely linked to sodium. When dietary sodium intake increases, serum levels of lithium are likely to decrease because lithium is excreted more rapidly. Conversely, when sodium in the diet decreases or when sodium is lost in ways other than through the kidney (e.g., sweating or diarrhea), serum lithium levels increase. Because a therapeutic serum level of lithium is not much lower than a toxic serum level, such considerations are significant. Also, diet and activity levels should not change abruptly in patients who are prescribed lithium. Lithium may produce nephrogenic diabetes insipidus, with resulting polyuria and polydipsia. Because of its pronounced effects in impairing the urine-concentrating effects of the kidney, patients taking lithium may void 3 liters per day or more. This may result in volume depletion or electrolyte imbalances as well as potentially worsen preexisting urinary incontinence.

Drug Interactions

Drugs that can elevate lithium serum levels include diuretics, which increase sodium excretion or decrease lithium excretion, thereby elevating serum lithium levels. Although thiazide diuretics are most commonly reported to cause increased lithium levels, other diuretics may produce this effect. To avoid this problem, reducing the dose of lithium by one-third if a diuretic is added is reasonable, with frequent checking of lithium levels for several weeks. Angiotensin-converting enzyme inhibitors have been reported to increase lithium levels by 36% (Finley et al. 1996). Indomethacin and other nonsteroidal anti-inflammatory drugs (NSAIDs) may increase serum lithium levels by reducing renal elimination, although sulindac may be somewhat less likely to do so (Lenox and Manji 1995). Some drugs decrease serum lithium levels and pose problems of inadequate treatment and symptom exacerbation. This decrease may occur in one of two ways: by increasing lithium excretion or by decreasing lithium absorption. Drugs that increase lithium excretion include acetazolamide, caffeine, and alcohol.

Using Lithium

Lithium is well absorbed from the gastrointestinal tract and is normally given in oral tablets, capsules, or concentrates. Peak serum levels are reached in 1–4 hours. More than 95% of the amount ingested is excreted by the kidneys (i.e., not metabolized). The plasma half-life is approximately 24 hours. Lithium, an ion interchangeable with sodium, has a variety of physiological and pathophysiological actions in various organs. It is important to ascertain whether the patient has any medical contraindications to lithium, especially renal impairment. Patients on low-salt diets or taking diuretics should have their electrolyte values determined. A baseline electrocardiogram (ECG) is necessary to rule out preexisting arrhythmia or nodal block. Lithium can produce repolarization changes in the ECG (ST segment and T wave), and 20% of patients develop a flattened T wave or inversion at therapeutic blood levels not indicating underlying heart disease. Before initiating lithium, baseline laboratory studies consisting of a complete blood count (CBC), electrolytes, blood urea nitrogen (BUN), creatinine, T4, thyroid-stimulating hormone, and urinalysis should be performed. A baseline 24-hour creatinine clearance is useful but difficult to obtain in an agitated patient. Review of current medications is mandatory; if possible, diuretics and NSAIDs should be discontinued.

Lithium is usually started at a dose of 150 mg once or twice daily. The dosage may be increased by 150 mg/day in 3 or 4 days, and a serum level should then be checked within 4 days. Further dosage increases may be needed to obtain a serum level of between 0.4 and 0.8 mEq/L. Serum levels are then checked several times after a dosage increase to ensure that the patient is indeed at steady state, after which lithium levels can be obtained every 2–4 months for most patients. For some patients who receive concomitant medications that may increase lithium levels, it may be prudent to check monthly lithium levels. If any new side effects emerge, such as confusion, ataxia, or gastrointestinal side effects, lithium and serum electrolyte levels should be obtained. Patients or their caregivers need to be educated on the signs and symptoms of lithium toxicity as well as the need to maintain an adequate intake of water and salt. They must also be advised on an avoidance of diuretics, NSAIDs, and angiotensin-converting enzyme inhibitors without notification of the physician prescribing the lithium.

Carbamazepine

Clinical studies and case reports of the use of carbamazepine in this population have frequently included the concomitant use of other active medications. Thus, interpretation of reports using carbamazepine is difficult with respect to carbamazepine's "pure" effect. Clearly, carbamazepine is effective in patients with bipolar disorder. Six controlled studies, one of which was placebo controlled, have shown carbamazepine's efficacy. However, in our clinical experience, the use of carbamazepine for agitation often requires the addition of an adjunctive agent or agents. Also, carbamazepine is associated with more serious adverse effects than some of the other mood-stabilizing agents discussed below.

Compared with lithium, carbamazepine has received more attention in treating dementia associated with agitation. Carbamazepine was one of the first investigated mood stabilizers to be used for agitation and aggression and is currently used for those with a variety of syndromes (e.g., head injury and alcoholic encephalopathy). Possible mechanisms for its use include stabilization of limbic kindling phenomenon, direct neurochemical effects, and antidepressant and antimanic effects. A number of uncontrolled studies (Chambers et al. 1982; Essa 1986; Gleason and Schneider 1994; Leibovici and Tariot 1988; Lemke 1995; Marin and Greenwald 1990; Patterson 1987, 1988; Schneider et al. 1989; Tariot et al. 1995, 1998) have reported on carbamazepine's positive and specific effects on aggression, agitation, mood, and affective lability. These studies show a robust effect of carbamazepine versus placebo or baseline clinical measures. Carbamazepine is most useful in cases with temporal lobe electroencephalogram (EEG) abnormalities. Patients with psychosis or excitability may also benefit from carbamazepine with or without adjunctive antipsychotic agents. In their excellent review, Schneider and Sobin (1991) summarized six open-label studies of carbamazepine that involved 29 patients, 25 of whom showed a significant response, as well as one controlled trial that showed no significant effect of carbamazepine. In a placebo-controlled study of 51 nursing home patients with agitation and dementia, Tariot et al. (1998) found that 77% of patients receiving carbamazepine improved on the Clinical Global Impression scale (Guy 1976), compared with 21% of patients receiving placebo. The mean daily dosage was 304 mg/day, and the mean serum level was 5.3 μg/mL. Carbamazepine was well tolerated in a population that the authors described as "old, frail, medically complex, severely demented, and functionally impaired," with only one patient in the carbamazepine group dropping out because of side effects (Tariot el al. 1998). In a prior study, Tariot et al. (1995) administered carbamazepine or placebo to 25 nursing home patients with dementia in double-blind, crossover fashion and found that a modal dosage of 300 mg/day was tolerated with a mean serum level of 5.7 μg/mL. No significant differences were found in side effects between placebo and carbamazepine. Clinically insignificant elevations of alkaline phosphatase, alanine aminotransferase, and gamma-glutamyl transferase were seen after 5 weeks of treatment.

Side Effects

The most commonly reported side effects of carbamazepine are ataxia, drowsiness, gastrointestinal upset, weight gain, and leukopenia. Carbamazepine can also cause aplastic anemia, which is reported to occur in 1 in 20,000 to 1 in 125,000 patients and is unrelated to the transient, benign leukopenia more commonly observed (McDonald and Nemeroff 1996). Other reported side effects are hyponatremia, blurred vision or diplopia, rash, and elevation of liver enzymes. Because carbamazepine has been associated with Stevens-Johnson syndrome, a rash appearing in a patient treated with carbamazepine should be investigated. McElroy and Keck (1995) advise that as long as no fever, bleeding, exfoliative skin lesions, or other signs of hypersensitivity are seen, carbamazepine may be continued despite the appearance of a rash. Rare, idiosyncratic side effects, including pancreatitis, hepatic failure, and bradycardia, may also be seen (McElroy and Keck 1995).

Drug Interactions

Carbamazepine induces the cytochrome P450 enzyme system and may cause a reduction in coadministered antipsychotic agents, prednisone, theophylline, warfarin, or valproate (McElroy and Keck 1995). Conversely, nefazodone, diltiazem, verapamil, propoxyphene, and erythromycin may cause carbamazepine toxicity if used together because they inhibit metabolism of carbamazepine. Carbamazepine is also highly protein bound, and levels may increase if coadministered with aspirin, digoxin, or selective serotonin reuptake inhibitors (SSRIs) (McDonald and Nemeroff 1996).

Using Carbamazepine

A pretreatment workup should include a CBC with differential, electrolytes, and liver function tests. Because of its structural similarity to the tricyclic antidepressants (TCAs), obtaining an ECG before initiating carbamazepine is desirable, but it is not routinely done. The dosage should be initiated at 100 mg twice a day and increased by 100 mg/day every 3 or 4 days as tolerated. After a patient has been taking 400 mg/day for 4 days, a serum level can be drawn, and the dose can be titrated to maintain a level between 4 and 12 µg/mL. Weekly CBC and liver function tests for the first 4 weeks are recommended by some authors (McDonald and Nemeroff 1996), after which a CBC should be obtained monthly for several months and then checked every 3–6 months indefinitely. Periodic monitoring of liver function tests (e.g., every 3–6 months) is also reasonable. Carbamazepine should be discontinued if the neutrophil count drops below 500, liver function tests increase to more than twice their baseline values, or total white blood cell count drops below 2,500. Despite this surveillance, life-threatening blood dyscrasias, hepatic failure, or exfoliative dermatitis may occur. The best prevention is adequate education of the family and other caregivers about signs and symptoms of hepatic, hematological, and dermatological symptoms to watch for (e.g., anorexia, abdominal pain, easy bruising, sore throat).

Valproate

Valproate, like lithium and carbamazepine, has demonstrated efficacy in treating mania associated with bipolar disorder. Valproate (divalproex sodium or Depakote) has gained significant popularity in the treatment of patients with acute and chronic agitation. In this regard, the quality of clinical reports is certainly better than that found with other mood-stabilizing drugs. Valproate appears to be effective in cases in which mood cycling is associated with agitation and appears to be superior in situations in which dysphoria is a prominent clinical feature (Keltner and Folks, 1997). Moreover, valproate is generally better tolerated than lithium and other mood-stabilizing agents and may be uniquely effective in patients who exhibit rapid mood cycling. A comorbid condition that may prompt its use is posttraumatic stress disorder; the agent may also be used in patients with associated psychotic syndromes (Wilcox 1994). Open trials and chart reviews have shown that agitation and aggression in dementia are quite responsive with respect to baseline evaluations. Mellow et al. (1993) were the first to report divalproex's tolerability, in a 1- to 3-month trial in four patients. Dosages in this study ranged from 750 to 2,500 mg/day with blood levels ranging from 45 to 93 µg/mL. In another study, Lott et al. (1995) treated 10 nursing home patients with dementia and behavioral agitation with doses of 375–750 mg/day for up to 34 weeks. Eight of 10 patients showed a significant reduction in the frequency of episodes of agitation. Moreover, this response was maintained in all patients, with minimal side effects and excellent tolerability. Puryear et al. (1995) reported that 12 of 13 elderly patients, most of whom had bipolar disorder, tolerated valproate well with a mean daily dose of 1,000 mg and a mean serum level of 57 ng/mL. Other studies using divalproex sodium have consistently reported positive findings (Horne and Lindley 1995; Porsteinsson et al. 1997; Sandborn et al. 1995; Sival et al. 1994).

Side Effects

Valproate can produce anorexia, nausea, dyspepsia, diarrhea, tremors, weight gain, alopecia, and sedation (McElroy and Keck 1995). Benign elevation of transaminase levels and transient thrombocytopenia can also occur. Because of the latter, it is desirable to avoid aspirin while taking valproate (McDonald and Nemeroff 1996).

Drug Interactions

Unlike carbamazepine, valproate inhibits hepatic enzymes and thus slows metabolism of other drugs such as phenobarbital, phenytoin, and TCAs.

Because of the complex interactions, pharmacokinetics, and pharmacody-namics of valproate and carbamazepine, this combination may be prob-lematic; however, some studies suggest that this combination may be well tolerated and very effective in severely agitated and aggressive patients with dementia (Keltner and Folks 1997). Valproate levels may be de-creased by the coadministration of carbamazepine because of the latter's tendency to increase microsomal enzyme activity. As with carbamazepine, valproate is highly protein-bound and should be used with caution in pa-tients receiving other highly protein-bound drugs. Lithium in combina-tion with divalproex may also be used. However, the combination is more likely to produce moderate to severe adverse side effects; these side effects tend to be associated with lithium.

Using Valproate

Valproate and related compounds have been used since the 1960s as anti-epileptic agents. The various formulations of valproate differ with respect to absorption and potential side effects. Formulations such as Depekane are rapidly absorbed in 2 hours or less, but divalproex (Depakote) in the form of an enteric-coated or "sprinkle" tablet is more slowly absorbed, in 4 hours or more. Common side effects include gastrointestinal upset, somnolence, tremor, and dizziness. These dose-related side effects can be avoided or minimized by using the enteric-coated formulation or sprinkle tablet. Be-fore starting the drug, a CBC, platelet count, and liver function tests should be obtained. Valproate should be started at 125–250 mg twice daily, and the dose increased by 125–250 mg/day every 2–3 days. A reasonable target dosage is 500 mg/day, at which time a serum level can be checked. Thera-peutic dosages are from 15 to 20 mg/kg/day. A more rapid titration sched-ule for severe agitation and aggressive behavior is often well tolerated. The target dosage is 15–20 mg/kg. For example, for a 164-pound (75-kg) per-son, start with 250 mg three times a day, then titrate to 250 mg three times a day and 500 mg at bedtime. If tolerated, advance to 500 mg three times a day. Generally, therapeutic levels occur between 50 and 120 µg/mL, which may be used to guide optimum therapeutic dose. The authors obtain a platelet count and liver function tests approximately every 2–4 weeks for the first 2 months of treatment. After that time, a valproate level, platelet count, and liver function tests should be checked every 3–6 months.

Gabapentin

Gabapentin was approved in early 1994 for antiepileptic use as an adjunc-tive treatment for partial seizures in adults and adolescents. The drug is similar to GABA in structure but with molecular alterations that make it more lipophilic and thus better able to penetrate the blood–brain barrier (Ramsey 1993). Its anticonvulsant effects appear unrelated to the GABA system.

Because other anticonvulsant agents have shown efficacy in treating agitation associated with brain damage, gabapentin has been used for this indication. Stanton et al. (1997) and others have found gabapentin useful in patients with such diverse problems as bipolar disorder, alcohol dependence, and bilateral frontal lobe injury whose presentation was primarily manic. Ryback and Ryback (1995) reported the successful use of gabapentin in an adolescent with closed head injury complicated by partial seizure disorder and intermittent explosive disorder. Gabapentin 1,200 mg/day (plus imipramine 150 mg/day) resulted in decreased frequency and intensity of explosive outbursts. Such findings suggest its potential use in agitated patients with dementia. Regan and Gordon (1997) reported a case of a 68-year-old agitated patient with dementia who exhibited violence toward the nursing home staff. She did not respond to buspirone, fluoxetine, trazadone, or haloperidol; gabapentin (300 mg twice daily plus haloperidol 2 mg at bedtime) significantly improved her behavior and cooperation with activities of daily living. Her family felt comfortable taking her for short drives, which they were previously unable to do so because of her irritability and severe agitation. Ultimately, her haloperidol dosage was reduced to 0.5 mg/day.

Side Effects

Gabapentin is usually well tolerated. Reported side effects have included somnolence, dizziness, ataxia, fatigue, and nystagmus (Andrews and Fischer 1994; Olin 1995). Because gabapentin is not hepatically metabolized and is excreted unchanged by the kidneys, it has little potential for pharmacokinetic drug–drug interactions. For example, it can be coadministered with carbamazepine or divalproex with little or no effect on blood levels of these other agents.

Drug Interactions

Gabapentin has no drug interactions with other antiepileptic drugs. Antacids reduce its bioavailability, and cimetidine increases it.

Using Gabapentin

Because gabapentin is renally excreted unchanged, it is desirable to check renal function tests before a patient starts receiving the drug. The usual starting dosage in younger adults is 300 mg/day with the addition of 300 mg/day every day until a dose of 300 mg three times a day is reached. Although there are no guidelines specific to dosing in geriatric patients, the package insert gives clear guidelines for maximum daily dose based on creatinine clearance. We initiate the drug at 100 mg once or twice a day and increase the dosage by 100 mg/day every 2 or 3 days. In the absence of renal impairment, a daily dose of approximately 600–1,200 mg is reasonable in divided doses, based on clinical response. Absorption of gabapentin is dose dependent at high dosages. Food does not alter absorption. Gabapentin has a relatively short half-life of 5–8 hours. It is not protein bound to any extent, and it is not measurably metabolized; thus, it is excreted as an unchanged molecule in urine. Patients with decreased renal function should be given smaller doses. Therapeutic serum levels, which are not routinely obtained, are approximately greater than 2 µg/mL.

Lamotrigine

Lamotrigine was approved in late 1994 as an adjunctive treatment for patients with partial seizures and may have implications for more generalized seizures in the future. It is related to the antifolate compound pyrimidine. It blocks sustained repetitive firing of neurons by prolonging the inactivation of sodium channels in animal models, and it may be by this mechanism that it suppresses seizure activity (Meldrum 1994). Lamotrigine is thought to have some mood-stabilizing properties. This agent also has inhibitory effects on the excitatory neurotransmitter glutamate, which may explain its mechanism of action in the treatment of bipolar disorder and other related disorders. Currently, there are no reports of lamotrigine's use in treating agitation associated with dementia, but it is likely that case reports will be forthcoming. Indeed, in an open, prospective, 12-month trial involving 67 treatment-refractory bipolar patients, Calabrese et al. (1995) found a broad spectrum of efficacy. Lamotrigine seems to have both antidepressant and antimanic effects with respect to mood cycling and rapid cycling patients. A number of open trials have reported generally positive results in bipolar patients (reviewed in Pollack and Scott 1997). Thus, lamotrigine at 50–250 mg/day may have benefit in agitated patients with dementia and associated mood disturbances. An additional consideration may be patients with dementia who exhibit self-injurious behavior. One uncontrolled case report suggested that lamotrigine was useful in the treatment of self-injurious behavior, which has been linked with excessive glutaminergic activity in animal models (Davanzo and King 1996).

Side Effects

Lamotrigine is associated with the development of rash in about 10% of cases, and severe Stevens-Johnson type syndromes may occur in about 0.1% of adults. Lamotrigine should be discontinued in any patient who develops a rash. More benign side effects include dizziness, ataxia, somnolence, headache, and double vision. The induction of mania may turn out to be a limiting side effect of lamotrigine in some patients, but antidepressant effects look quite promising.

Drug Interactions

Lamotrigine must be used with caution. With individuals taking a microsomal enzyme–inducing agent such as carbamazepine, phenytoin, phenobarbital, or primidone, use a starting dose of 25–50 mg once daily for 2 weeks, increasing by 25 mg/day for another 2 weeks, and then weekly increases of 25–50 mg/day to the usually therapeutic dosage of 150–400 mg in divided doses. It is important to note that valproate markedly increases the levels of lamotrigine and reduces its clearance. If valproate is being taken in combination, then the starting dose should be 12.5–25 mg every other day, with the titration occurring over a period that is twice as long.

Olanzapine

Olanzapine (Zyprexa) was approved in late 2000 for the treatment of acute mania associated with bipolar disorder, based on two placebo-controlled trials (Tohen et al. 1999, 2000). Recently presented data also support the efficacy of olanzapine as monotherapy in the treatment of the depressed phase of bipolar disorder (Tohen et al. 2002a). Based on these studies as well as evidence from a study comparing olanzapine with divalproex (Tohen et al. 2002b), it is evident that olanzapine stabilizes mood in many patients with bipolar disorder. Therefore, olanzapine is considered to be unique among the antipsychotics in possessing the necessary characteristics to justify being considered a mood stabilizing medication.

Olanzapine has been demonstrated to reduce agitation and aggression in patients with schizophrenia as well as in patients with dementia. Studies of olanzapine, specific to the reduction of acute and chronic agitation in the dementia population, are discussed elsewhere in this text (Chapter 12).

Side Effects

Olanzapine has been extensively studied in the elderly patient population. Its adverse effects pattern has been demonstated in the elderly to be very similar to that observed in young patients with the same underlying illnesses. Olanzapine can produce transient elevations in liver enzymes, sedation that is only rarely severe, changes in gait without evidence of a significant increase in falls when compared to placebo, and hypotension (particularly early in treatment when used in combination with benzodiazepines). Likely due to its antihistaminergic properties, olanzapine does produce dry mouth; possibly due to its serotonergic receptor antagonist effects, it also produces mild to moderate constipation in a small number of patients. In the dementia population, unlike other diagnostic groups, olanzapine produces only minimal averaged weight gain. Olanzapine does not not demonstrate the clinically significant ability to systematically alter cardiac conduction as indexed by such parameters as the corrected QT interval (QTc). As indicated in olanzapine's FDA-approved package insert, it should be used with caution—as with all centrally active medicines—in patients with dementia.

Drug Interactions

Olanzapine is not renally cleared; thus, dosing is not dependent on the patient's renal status. Olanzapine is preferentially metabolized through the P450-1a system, a pathway that is not subject to significant genetic variation. Co-administration studies of olanzapine with other medications metabolized by the P450-1a system, such as theophylline, indicate that olanzapine's interaction with the P450-1a enzymes is competitive and that olanzapine neither inhibits nor induces this pathway. Therefore, its use in patients who are taking medications or substances (such as caffeine) that also competively interact with this pathway would be expected to produce no clinically significant changes in the levels of either olanzapine or the other substance/medication. This is not the case for medications/substances that induce P450-1a enyme synthesis (such as nicotine). In this instance, olanzapine serum concentrations are reduced. Similarly, medications/substances that inhibit the activity of the P450-1a system (such as fluvoxamine) will produce elevated serum concentrations of olanzapine. However, the significance of elevated olanzapine serum concentrations is unlikely to be clinically important due to olanzapine's very wide therapeutic window. Olanzapine can be extensively metabolized by many P450 pathways other than P450-1a, including the P450-2D6 and P450-3A4 pathways. Therefore, if any one pathway becomes inhibited by a competing medication or substance, olanzapine metabolism flows over to any of several other available P450 system enzyme systems to be metabolized. In summary, P450-based drug–drug interactions are not a significant concern with olanzapine. As noted previously, drug–drug interactions that arise due to pharmacodynamic interactions are more likely to be observed. Such interactions include, for example, hypotension and additive sedation in co-use of olanzapine and benzodiazepines.

When to Use a Mood Stabilizer

Use of mood stabilizers in the treatment of patients with agitation can effectively control a wide range of behavioral disturbances, including aggression, combativeness, shouting, hyperactivity, and disinhibition. Certainly, patients who exhibit mood lability are excellent candidates for use of these particular agents. Successful use of mood stabilizers should aim to minimize behavioral disturbance, maximize functioning independence, and foster a safe and secure environment. To this end, it is useful to schedule regular patient surveillance and monitoring; work closely with the family and caregivers or clinical staff; establish programs to improve mood and behavior with activities; and encourage environmental modification to achieve moderate amounts of stimulation in the context of a nonthreatening, familiar environment (Small et al. 1997). Another consideration is whether the patient being treated has any evidence of seizure activity, such as an EEG with focal abnormalities, episodic unprovoked aggression, absence episodes, or unexplained lapses of consciousness. Certainly, in patients with known seizure disorders, dementia, and agitation, anticonvulsant agents may be used to treat seizures and agitation regardless of whether the two are etiologically related. In this situation, patients may already be receiving an anticonvulsant agent such as phenobarbital or phenytoin. Because these agents have less to support their role in treating agitation and are often poorly tolerated in elderly patients with dementia, it may be preferable to switch such patients to valproate or carbamazepine and possibly augment with gabapentin if needed to control breakthrough seizures or behavioral symptoms. When doing so, it is generally best to add the new anticonvulsant agent to the existing one, being mindful of potential pharmacokinetic interactions often seen when anticonvulsants are combined. After the new agent is at a therapeutic blood level, the old agent may be gradually tapered over several weeks. Frequent monitoring of blood levels of the new drug during the taper is necessary. Consultation with a neurologist may be required when seizure control is suboptimal.

Choosing a Mood Stabilizer

In patients with known or suspected seizures, the choice of a mood stabilizer is based on which agent is most likely to treat the patient's type of seizure. In other patients, however, the choice is made based on pharmacological properties, primarily the side effect profile, the potential for drug–drug interactions, the properties of other medications taken by the patient, and coexisting medical problems. For example, a patient with preexisting thrombocytopenia would probably not be a candidate for treatment with valproate, which can itself cause thrombocytopenia. Similarly, a patient with severe renal insufficiency but normal hepatic function would be better served with valproate than gabapentin. All other things being equal, our first choice of mood stabilizer is usually valproate, followed by gabapentin. We use carbamazepine less often, mostly because it seems to cause more ataxia than valproate and is more difficult to titrate. Because of its narrow therapeutic index, poor tolerability (even at therapeutic levels) in geriatric patients, and limited efficacy, we rarely use lithium in this population.

Combination Therapy

Generally, it is preferable to avoid combining mood stabilizers. However, in difficult-to-manage patients, combining valproate and gabapentin or carbamazepine and gabapentin may be of value. The strategy used in combination therapy is to add a second drug of a different class rather than switching agents. If the patient shows no response to a mood stabilizer, however, switching to a second makes more sense. As previously noted, valproate is the first-line choice in most cases because of its superior side effect profile and the ability to rapidly titrate to an effective dose. Combining valproate and carbamazepine should be reserved for patients with intractable agitation or those whose underlying seizure disorder might warrant such a combination. Combining a mood stabilizer with other psychotropic drugs (e.g., buspirone, antidepressants, or antipsychotics) may usually be safely done if moderate doses of both are used and levels of the mood stabilizer are monitored appropriately.

References

Andrews CO, Fischer JH: Gabapentin: a new agent for the management of epilepsy. Ann Pharmacotherapy 28:1188–1196, 1994
Arya DK: Lithium-induced neurotoxicity at serum lithium levels within the therapeutic range. Aust NZ J Psychiatry 30:871–873, 1996

Calabrese JR, Bowden CL, McElroy S, et al: Efficacy of lamotrigine in bipolar disorder: preliminary data. Presented at the Second International Conference on Affective Disorders. Jerusalem, Israel, September 1995

Casanova B, de Entrambasaguas M, Perla C, et al: Lithium-induced Creutzfeldt-Jakob syndrome. Clin Neuropharmacol 19:356–359, 1996

Chambers CA, Bain J, Rosbottom R, et al: Carbamazepine in senile dementia and over activity: a placebo controlled double blind trial. IRCS Medical Science 10:505–506, 1982

Davanzo PA, King BH: Open trial of lamotrigine in the treatment of self-injurious behavior in an adolescent with profound mental retardation. J Child Adolesc Psychopharmacol 6:273–279, 1996

Essa M: Carbamazepine in dementia. J Clin Psychopharmacol 6:234–236, 1986

Finley PR, O'Brien JG, Coleman RW: Lithium and angiotensin-converting enzyme inhibitors: evaluation of a potential interaction. J Clin Psychopharmacol 16:68–71, 1996

Gleason RP, Schneider LS: Carbamazepine treatment of nursing home patients with dementia: a preliminary study. J Am Geriatr Soc 42:1160–1166, 1994

Guy W (ed): ECDEU Assessment Manual for Psychopharmacology (DHEW Publ ADM 76-338). Rockville, MD, U.S. Dept of Health, Education and Welfare, 1976, pp 217–222

Holroyd S, Smith D: Disabling Parkinsonism due to lithium: a case report. J Geriatr Psychiatry Neurol 8:118–119, 1995

Horne M, Lindley SE: Divalproex sodium in the treatment of aggressive behavior and dysphoria in patients with organic brain syndromes. J Clin Psychiatry 56:430–431, 1995

Janicak PG, Davis JM, Preskorn SH, et al: Treatment with mood stabilizers/antimanics, in Principles and Practice of Psychopharmacotherapy. Baltimore, MD, Williams & Wilkins, 1993, pp 341–404

Keltner NL, Folks, DG: Mood disorders, in Handbook of Psychotropic Drugs, 2nd Edition. St. Louis, MO, CV Mosby, 1997, pp 80–128

Leibovici A, Tariot PN: Carbamazepine treatment of agitation associated with dementia. J Geriatr Psychiatry Neurol 1:110–112, 1988

Lemke MR: Effect of carbamazepine on agitation in Alzheimer's inpatients refractory to neuroleptics. J Clin Psychiatry 56:354–357, 1995

Lenox RH, Manji HK: Lithium, in The American Psychiatric Press Textbook of Psychopharmacology. Edited by Schatzberg AF, Nemeroff CB. Washington, DC, American Psychiatric Press, 1995, pp 303–349

Liptzin B: Treatment of mania, in Clinical Geriatric Psychopharmacology, 2nd Edition. Edited by Salzman C. Baltimore, MD, Williams & Wilkins, 1992, pp 177–190

Lott AD, McElroy SL, Keys MA: Valproate in the treatment of behavioral agitation in elderly patients with dementia. J Neuropsychiatry Clin Neurosci 7:314–319, 1995

Marin DB, Greenwald BS: Carbamazepine for aggressive agitation in demented patients during nursing care (letter). Am J Psychiatry 51:115–118, 1990

McDonald WM, Nemeroff CB: The diagnosis and treatment of mania in the elderly. Bull Menninger Clin 60:174–196, 1996

McElroy SL, Keck PE: Antiepileptic drugs, in The American Psychiatric Press Textbook of Psychopharmacology. Edited by Schatzberg AF, Nemeroff CB. Washington, DC, American Psychiatric Press, 1995, pp 351–375

Meldrum BS: Lamotrigine: a novel approach. Seizure 3(suppl A):41–45, 1994

Mellow AM, Solano-Lopez C, Davis S: Sodium valproate in the treatment of behavioral disturbance in dementia. J Geriatr Psychiatry Neurol 6:205–209, 1993

Olin BR, editor: Drug Facts and Comparisons. St. Louis, MO, Wolters Kluwer, 1995

Patterson JF: Carbamazepine for assaultive patients with organic brain disease. Psychosomatics 28:579–581, 1987

Patterson JF: A preliminary study of carbamazepine in the treatment of assaultive patients with dementia. J Geriatr Psychiatry Neurol 1:21–23, 1988

Pollack MH, Scott EL: Gabapentin and lamotrigine: novel treatments for mood and anxiety disorders. CNS Spectrums 10:56–61, 1997

Porsteinsson A, Tariot PN, Erb R, et al: An open trial of valproate for agitation in geriatric neuropsychiatric disorder. Am J Geriatr Psychiatry 5:344–351, 1997

Puryear LJ, Kunik ME, Workman R: Tolerability of divalproex sodium in elderly psychiatric patients with mixed diagnoses. J Geriatr Psychiatry Neurol 8:234–237, 1995

Ramsey RE: Clinical Issues in the Management of Epilepsy. Miami, FL, University of Miami Press, 1993

Regan WM, Gordon SM: Gabapentin for behavioral agitation in Alzheimer's disease (letter). J Clin Psychopharmacol 17:59–60, 1997

Ryback R, Ryback L: Gabapentin for behavioral dyscontrol (letter). Am J Psychiatry 152:1399, 1995

Sandborn WD, Bendfelt F, Hamdy R: Valproic acid for physically aggressive behavior in geriatric patients. Am J Geriatr Psychiatry 3:239–242, 1995

Schneider LS, Sobin PB: Non-neuroleptic medications in the management of agitation in Alzheimer's disease and other dementia: a selective review. Int J Geriatr Psychiatry 6:691–708, 1991

Schneider LS, Gleason RP, Chui HC: Progressive supranuclear palsy with agitation: response to trazodone but not to thiothixene or carbamazepine. J Geriatr Psychiatry Neurol 2:109–112, 1989

Sival R, Haffmans P, VanGent P, et al: The effect of sodium valproate on disturbed behavior in dementia. J Am Geriatr Soc 42:906–907, 1994

Small GW, Rabins PV, Barry RP, et al: Diagnosis and treatment of Alzheimer disease and related disorders: consensus statement of the American Association for Geriatric Psychiatry, the Alzheimer's Association, and the American Geriatrics Society. JAMA 2786:1363–1371, 1997

Stanton SP, Keck PE, McElroy SI: Treatment of acute mania with gabapentin (letter). Am J Psychiatry 154:287, 1997

Tariot PN, Frederiksen K, Erb R, et al: Lack of carbamazepine toxicity in frail nursing home patients: a controlled study. J Am Geriatr Soc 43:1026–1029, 1995

Tariot PN, Erb R, Podgorski CA, et al: Efficacy and tolerability of carbamazepine for agitation and aggression in dementia. Am J Psychiatry 155:54–61, 1998

Tohen M, Sanger TM, McElroy SL, et al: Olanzapine versus placebo in the treatment of acute mania. Am J Psychiatry 156:702–709, 1999

Tohen M, Jacobs TG, Grundy SL, et al: Efficacy of olanzapine in acute bipolar mania: a double-blind, placebo-controlled study. Arch Gen Psychiatry 57:841–849, 2000

Tohen M, Vieta E, Ketter T, et al: Olanzapine and olanzapine-fluoxetine combination (OFC) in the treatment of bipolar depression. Paper presented at the 155th annual meeting of the American Psychiatric Association, Philadelphia, PA, 2002a

Tohen M, Baker RW, Altshuler L, et al: Olanzapine versus divalproex for the treatment of acute mania. Am J Psychiatry 159:1011–1017, 2002b

Wilcox J: Divalproex sodium in the treatment of aggressive behavior. Ann Clin Psychiatry 6:17–20, 1994

CHAPTER 12

Antipsychotic Agents

David G. Folks, M.D.

Delusions, hallucinations, and disruptive behaviors with psychomotor agitation and physical aggression occur in 90% of the patients with dementia at some point during the course of the illness (Devanand et al. 1997; Reisberg et al. 1987; Rubin et al. 1987; Tariot 1996). Psychosis and disruptive behaviors are associated with a more rapidly dementing course (Drevets and Rubin 1989; Rosen and Zubenko 1991; Stern et al. 1987). Untreated psychoses and disruptive behaviors are also distressing to patients and caregivers (Small and Jarvik 1982) and more often lead to institutionalization (Haller et al. 1989; Rabins et al. 1982). Whereas psychomotor agitation occurs in nearly half of patients with dementia in outpatient clinics and long-term care facilities, aggressive behavior occurs less commonly (Cohen-Mansfield et al. 1989; Devanand et al. 1992; Swearer et al. 1988). The prevalence of delusions with dementia depends on the clinical setting, and ranges from 0%–50% (Reisberg et al. 1989). However, isolated symptoms (e.g., the belief that people are stealing things) are more common than are more typical psychotic disorders (Wragg and Jeste 1989). Hallucinations are rarely manifested early in the illness but increase in prevalence as dementia progresses.

A systematic approach to agitation with or without psychosis involves an initial evaluation of the patient to address underlying problems, including medical comorbidities, followed by nonpharmacological management and the choice of an appropriate medication with optimization of therapy through a process of trial and error. Antipsychotic agents are frequently prescribed for psychotic disorders as well as agitation and disruptive behavior in patients with dementia (Avorn et al. 1989; Devanand and Levy

167

1995). The use of antipsychotic agents is considered a first-line treatment in patients with psychosis and agitation with disruptive behavior.

Conventional or Typical Antipsychotic Agents

The first studies of antipsychotic agents in dementia used flawed research designs that included diagnostic heterogeneity and the use of concomitant psychotropic medications. Two of these earlier studies used placebo-controlled designs. Petrie et al. (1982) performed an 8-week study with haloperidol and loxapine using mean doses of 4.6 and 21.9 mg, respectively. Both drugs improved patient outcome when administered at relatively low doses, but side effects, sedation, and extrapyramidal symptoms (EPS) were increased over placebo. Using somewhat lower doses of loxapine and thioridazine, 10.5 and 62.5 mg, respectively, Barnes et al. (1982) showed that both medications as well as placebo were associated with behavioral improvements at the end of 8 weeks, with greater improvement observed for loxapine and thioridazine. Patients with more severe initial behavioral symptoms were more likely to improve with the antipsychotic agents versus placebo.

A meta-analysis of seven studies published from 1966 to 1989 suggested moderate superiority of antipsychotics over placebo in the treatment of psychosis and disruptive or agitated behaviors in dementia (Schneider et al. 1990). These studies compared antipsychotics with placebo, resulting in improvement of 41% for placebo versus 59% for drug ($P=0.004$). The effect size of the meta-analysis was reduced by the high placebo response rate in some of the studies (Barnes et al. 1982; Rada and Kellner 1976). Besides asserting "modest efficacy," no single antipsychotic agent was deemed better than another.

Since 1990, surprisingly few studies have been conducted with typical antipsychotic drugs in patients with dementia. Carlyle et al. (1993) conducted a trial of loxapine versus haloperidol, 36 and 7 mg, respectively. Both agents were equally effective in reducing agitation and aggression, with fewer side effects noted for loxapine. A double-blind comparison of zuclopenthixol and thioridazine yielded equally significant improvements in both groups, with better effect on sleep disturbance from zuclopenthixol. This study was consistent with previous findings that low-potency, highly anticholinergic antipsychotic agents do not appear to cause more side effects than do higher potency antipsychotic agents. Another double-blind, placebo-controlled trial examined thiothixene in 36 agitated nursing home patients with dementia (Finkel et al. 1995). Significant improvement in agitation scores in 65% of thiothixene-treated patients were observed, compared with only 19% for placebo-treated patients. Other than sedation, no differences in treatment-emergent side effects were identified. Finally, Devanand et al. (1998) conducted a randomized, placebo-controlled, dose-comparison trial of haloperidol for psychoses and disruptive behaviors in patients with Alzheimer's disease (AD). The therapeutic effects were greater with the standard dosages of haloperidol (i.e., 2–3 mg/day) than with either the lower dosages or placebo. However, a subgroup developed moderate to severe EPS with higher dosages. A starting dosage of 1 mg/day with gradual upward dose titration was therefore recommended. The narrow therapeutic window observed with haloperidol may apply to other antipsychotic agents, consistent with the flexible dose study of thiothixene (Finkel et al. 1995).

Clinical Use of Conventional or Typical Antipsychotics

Behaviors unlikely to respond to a pharmacological treatment with conventional antipsychotics include wandering, pacing, and exit seeking. Screaming; inappropriate verbalizing (e.g., using foul language); resistance with toileting; inappropriate voiding, defecation, or spitting; inappropriate sexual behaviors (e.g., public masturbation); or disrobing are frequently not responsive to pharmacological intervention with antipsychotic agents (Schneider et al. 1990).

Behaviors that are more likely to respond to a pharmacological approach with antipsychotics include disorders involving coexisting Axis I psychiatric syndromes, especially psychosis, intermittent explosive disorder, or sleep cycle disruption (including sundowning syndrome) (Verma et al. 1998). The efficacy of conventional antipsychotics does not appear to be influenced by the choice of the specific antipsychotic drug. Low doses are considered as effective as higher doses and produce fewer side effects. Many patients who have participated in trials involving typical (or atypical) antipsychotics have manifested both psychoses and disruptive behaviors or agitation, making it difficult to evaluate whether antipsychotics are more specific for the treatment of psychotic features versus nonpsychotic agitation or disruptive behaviors (Raskind et al. 1987). Overall, conventional antipsychotics significantly reduce target symptoms that include hallucinations, delusions, paranoia, and excessive suspiciousness; however, the magnitude of effect on agitation and disruptive behaviors varies greatly. Larger samples are needed to evaluate whether the presence of specific subtypes of symptoms predict preferentially good response to antipsychotic treatment. Overall, the use of haloperidol 2–3 mg/day or equivalent doses of other antipsychotics leads to an acceptable trade-off between efficacy and side effects for dementia patients with psychosis and disruptive behaviors (Devanand et al. 1998).

The adverse effects of conventional antipsychotic agents in geriatric patients include orthostatic hypotension, which may result in falls and fractures; delirium; acute EPS; and autonomic dysfunction accompanied by urinary retention, constipation, or acute glaucoma (Avorn et al. 1994; Zarate et al. 1997). Geriatric patients with cognitive impairment are prone to antipsychotic-induced neurological side effects, particularly EPS. Long-term treatment is associated with the risk of developing tardive dyskinesia (TD) or (less often) neuroleptic malignant syndrome (Jeste et al. 1993).

General principles for the use of antipsychotic drugs in patients with dementia and agitation include starting with a low dose, going slow, and increasing only if necessary. Target symptoms, as previously mentioned, and side effects, including effects on cognition and activities of daily living, should be identified and assessed serially during antipsychotic treatment. The choice of antipsychotic depends more on the likelihood of adverse effect than on the differential efficacy. Nonresponse or intolerable side effects should lead to a dosage adjustment or a switch to an alternative antipsychotic or an alternative medication such as valproate or trazodone. No study has demonstrated a consistent advantage in the efficacy of one conventional antipsychotic over another. Haloperidol is among the most frequently prescribed agents in this category, but it does have a substantially higher incidence of EPS. Thiothixene, perphenazine, and loxapine are commonly used, but low-potency drugs such as chlorpromazine and thioridazine are more often avoided. A comparison of conventional antipsychotics is noted in Tables 12–1 and 12–2.

Atypical Antipsychotic Agents

Although conventional antipsychotics have remained the mainstay for the treatment of behavioral complications in dementia, newer, atypical antipsychotics possess a decreased propensity for EPS and related side effects and are becoming popular (Zarate et al. 1997). Atypical agents may be divided into three categories: 1) the relatively pure dopamine antagonists; 2) the dopamine D_2 serotonin 5-HT$_2$ norepinephrine antagonists (e.g., risperidone, ziprasidone, and sertindole); and 3) the multireceptor antagonists (e.g., clozapine, olanzapine, and quetiapine) (Table 12–3). Clozapine is still the most potent antipsychotic agent; olanzapine and seroquel represent the further development of clozapine's positive qualities; and risperidone and ziprasidone are dominated to a greater extent by relatively traditional dopamine D_2 receptor blockade.

Table 12–1. Comparison of selected antipsychotic agents: formulations, equivalent dosages, and relative side effects

Drug	Formulations	Approximate equivalent dose, mg	Degree of sedation	Anticholinergic effect	Orthostatic hypotension	Extrapyramidal symptoms
Chlorpromazine	Tablets, liquid, injection	100	High	Moderate	High	Moderate
Fluphenazine	Tablets, liquid, injection	2	Low	Low	Low	High
Haloperidol	Tablets, liquid, injection	2	Low	Low	Low	High
Loxapine	Capsules, liquid, injection	15	Moderate	Low	Moderate	Moderate
Mesoridazine	Tablets, liquid, injection	50	High	High	Moderate	Low
Molindone	Tablets, liquid	10	Low	Low	Low	Moderate
Perphenazine	Tablets, liquid, injection	10	Moderate	Low	Low	Moderate
Thioridazine	Tablets, liquid	100	High	High	High	Low
Thiothixene	Capsules, liquid, injection	5	Low	Low	Low	High
Trifluoperazine	Tablets, liquid, injection	5	Low	Low	Low	High

Source. Adapted from Keltner and Folks 1997.

Table 12-2. Receptor-binding profiles, clinical doses for agitation, and side effects of selected conventional antipsychotic agents

	Receptor binding						Clinical dose		Side effects		
	D_1	D_2	5-HT$_2$	Alpha-1	Anti-chol	Hist	Starting, mg/day	Typical, mg/day	Sedation	Autonomic	EPS
Haloperidol	–	+++	+	+	–	–	0.25–0.5	1–3	+	+	+++
Fluphenazine	–	+++	+	+	–	–	0.25–0.5	1–3	+	+	+++
Zuclopenthixol*	+	+++	+	++	–	–	N/A	N/A	++	++	++
Perphenazine	–	+++	++	++	–	++	2–4	8–16	++	+(+)	++
Thioridazine	+(+)	+++	++	+++	++	+	10–25	50–100	++(+)	++(+)	+
Chlorpromazine	–	+++	++	+++	++	++	12.5	50–100	+++	++(+)	+

Note.   –=negligible; +=mild; ++=moderate; +++=strong. Anti-chol= anticholinergic; EPS=extrapyramidal symptoms; Hist=histaminergic.
*Not available in United States.
Source.   Adapted from Keltner and Folks 1997; Gerlach and Peacock 1995.

Table 12-3. Receptor-binding profiles, clinical doses for agitation, and side effects of new atypical antipsychotic agents

	Receptor binding						Clinical dose		Side effects		
	D_1	D_2	5-HT$_2$	Alpha-1	Anti-chol	Hist	Starting, mg/day	Typical, mg/day	Sedation	Autonomic	EPS
D_2 antagonists											
Sulpiride*	–	+++	–	–	–	–	N/A	N/A	+	+	++
Amisulpiride*	–	+++	–	–	–	–	N/A	N/A	+	+	++
D_2–5-HT$_2$-alpha-1 antagonists											
Risperidone	–	+++	+++	+++	–	–	0.25–5.0	1–3	+	++	+
Ziprasidone*	+	+++	+++	++	–	–	10–20	20–80	++	++	++
Sertindole*	–	+	+++	++	–	–	N/A	N/A	+	++	+
Multireceptor antagonists											
Clozapine	++	++	+++	+++	+++	++	12.5	25–400	+++	+++	(+)
Olanzapine	++	+++	+++	++	–	++	1.25–2.5	2.5–15	++	+(+)	+
Quetiapine	(+)	+	+	+++	–	++	12.5–25	50–400	++	++	+

Note. – =negligible; + =mild; + + =moderate; + + + =strong. Anti-chol= anticholinergic; EPS=extrapyramidal symptoms; Hist=histaminergic.
*Not available in United States.
Source. Adapted from Keltner and Folks 1997; Gerlach and Peacock 1995.

Atypical antipsychotic agents offer significant theoretical advantages over conventional antipsychotics because of the reduced potential for EPS in a highly vulnerable population. These agents, especially clozapine, may cause orthostatic hypotension, with an increased risk of falls. Clozapine use in older patients with dementia is limited by the significantly greater potential for sedation: risperidone, olanzapine and quetiapine are better tolerated; sedation may occur when treatment is initiated, but tends to diminish with their continued use. Risperidone and quetiapine are more sedating than olanzapine but less sedating than clozapine. Of the four atypical antipsychotics currently available, risperidone has the highest incidence of EPS. From a theoretical perspective, antipsychotics such as clozapine with prominent anticholinergic properties may worsen cognition, but, as previously mentioned, anticholinergic side effects with thioridazine have not been empirically observed (Tune et al. 1992). Nonetheless, long-term therapeutic trials of acetylcholinesterase inhibitors in patients with AD have been associated with an incidental finding of improvement in disruptive behaviors (Raskind et al. 1997; Cummings 2001). Clearly, comparison of the relative efficacy and propensity for side effects of different classes of antipsychotics and other agents requires head-to-head controlled trials in patients with dementia and agitation (Devanand et al. 1998).

Clozapine

Clozapine, a dibenzodiazepine derivative, is an atypical antipsychotic agent that is characterized by marked antiadrenergic, antihistaminergic, antiserotonergic, and anticholinergic effects, with special affinity for dopamine D_4 receptors (Baldessarini et al. 1991; Meltzer 1991). Clozapine, with its therapeutic superiority, low level of EPS, and low dopamine D_2 and D_1 receptor occupancies at clinically effective doses, is the quintessential atypical antipsychotic, the standard against which new antipsychotics can be tested. However, the fact that it occupies a number of known receptors also results in a large number of side effects that pose serious problems for geriatric patients. Because of the risk of agranulocytosis, the use of clozapine is restricted to patients with unmanageable EPS, including TD or those who fail to respond to two or more traditional D_2-blocking antipsychotics. Although the risk of granulopenia and agranulocytosis are of utmost concern, the major side effects are sedation, hypersalivation, weight gain, orthostatic hypotension, and constipation.

Clozapine is effective at low doses (i.e., 50–200 mg) in treating patients with agitation and associated psychosis. EPS, bradykinesia, rigidity, and tremor occur less frequently or not at all with lower doses (Chacko et al. 1993; Salzman et al. 1995). Clozapine acts selectively on limbic dopamine receptors, with low affinity for the striatum and minimal effects on plasma prolactin levels. Thus, treatment-resistant patients with mood disorders or cognitive impairment with agitation may respond robustly to clozapine (Oberholzer et al. 1992). Possible mechanisms for clozapine's effect in patients with these conditions include the limbic D_4 receptors and anti-kindling antiadrenergic and antiserotonergic effects (Graham and Kokkinid-s 1993; Meltzer 1989). A substantial body of literature has demonstrated that clozapine is useful in the treatment of patients with Parkinson's disease who have agitated dementia (Nacasch et al. 1998).

Risperidone

Risperidone has shown significant promise in reducing psychotic and disruptive behaviors associated with dementia. Risperidone, a benzisoxazole derivative, is an atypical antipsychotic drug with high affinity and antagonistic action at serotonin 5-HT_2 receptors as well as D_2 dopamine receptors and considerable noradrenergic alpha-1 blockade. Lower doses of 1–2 mg clearly have advantages in relation to EPS, but higher doses approach similar side effects to conventional, high-potency antipsychotic agents. Compared with clozapine, risperidone offers the advantages of fewer anticholinergic symptoms and far less sedation, two important features to be considered in the selection of a drug.

Risperidone, compared with other atypical agents, has been more extensively studied in patients with dementia. One series, which involved 11 geriatric inpatients, noted remarkable improvement with risperidone despite adverse effects that included orthostasis, dizziness, abdominal cramps, headache, somnolence, and hypotension (Madhusoodanan et al. 1995). Herrmann et al. (1998) studied a series of 22 patients with dementia and behavioral disturbances including agitation, aggression, delusions, and hallucinations. Risperidone in dosages of 1–2 mg was well tolerated; 50% of the patients experienced significant improvement, although 50% experienced some EPS. Goldberg and Goldberg (1997) followed 109 patients with dementia-related behavioral disturbance over 6 months. Most initially received 0.25–0.5 mg of risperidone twice daily. Through questionnaires and clinical observation, these authors suggested that risperidone was well tolerated. Another study involved 625 nursing home patients and compared risperidone 0.5–2 mg with placebo for 12 weeks. Psychosis and aggression were significantly reduced with active drug ($P<0.05$), and a lower incidence of EPS below 2 mg was observed (Katz et al. 1999).

Meco et al. (1994) found that risperidone reduced or eliminated hallucinations without worsening EPS in L-dopa–treated patients with Parkinson's disease. Workman et al. (1997) conducted a pilot study that evaluated the effectiveness and tolerability of risperidone for the treatment of psychosis and agitation in nine patients with dementia, agitation, and Parkinson's disease. Interestingly, these investigators found risperidone to be effective and safe without worsening EPS or further impairing cognition. Lee et al. (1994) noted improvement in paranoia, hallucinations, and agitation with 2-mg doses of risperidone in dementia-associated aggression in Lewy body dementia. Deyn and Katz (2000) have described the utility of risperidone in aggression at low doses of 1–2 mg. Allen et al. (1995) described three additional patients with Lewy body dementia whose psychosis and agitation improved marketing with risperidone 0.5 mg once or twice daily. None of these patients declined in cognition, a concern noted with conventional antipsychotic agents in Lewy body dementia (Herrmann and Lanctot 1997).

Olanzapine, Quetiapine, and Ziprasidone

Olanzapine has a similar receptor binding profile to that of clozapine although a slightly higher affinity to all receptor sites except alpha-1 receptors. Significant side effects include dizziness, constipation, dry mouth, somnolence, agitation, asthenia, and nervousness. A placebo-controlled study by Street et al. (2000) established the optimal dosages at 5–10 mg for agitation, aggression, and psychosis. Another trial in nursing home patients found reduced symptoms of agitation and psychosis (Clark et al. 2001). Additionally, in this trial, patients were significantly less likely to develop psychosis while being treated with olanzapine. In my experience, olanzapine 1.25–15 mg/day has yielded significantly positive results in patients with agitated dementia.

Quetiapine is a strong alpha-1 receptor blocker with moderate antihistaminergic effect, weak dopamine D_2 serotonin 5-HT_2 antagonism, and very slight antagonism of dopamine D_1 receptors. Quetiapine possesses a very beneficial EPS profile and is generally more sedating than risperidone or olanzapine. In patients with schizophrenia, quetiapine has compared favorably to haloperidol at higher doses (i.e., 600 vs. 20 mg) (Emsley et al. 2001). However, lower dosages are used in patients with dementia. In my experience, 50–400 mg/day of quetiapine may yield significantly positive effects. Side effects include somnolence, dizziness, orthostatic hypotension, or lower blood pressure.

Ziprasidone is similar to risperidone in its receptor binding characteristics with a high ratio of 5-HT_2 to dopamine binding and noradrenergic to alpha-1 affinity. Ziprasidone has some affinity for 5-HT$_{1A}$ and D$_1$ receptors; this mechanism of action may potentially benefit patients with coexistent affective symptoms. Major side effects include sedation, nausea, headache, agitation, and dizziness. These adverse effects are much fewer with significantly less EPS compared with haloperidol.

Guidelines for Using Antipsychotic Agents in Agitated Dementia

Acute and Long-Term Treatment

Conventional high-potency antipsychotic agents such as haloperidol are ideal for treating acute-onset agitation in the context of delirium or for episodes of agitation requiring intramuscular administration. Intramuscular formulations of atypical antipsychotic agents, including depot forms, are under development but are not yet available. Antipsychotic agents are preferable for acute-onset severe agitation associated with aggression, anger, or sundowning. The drug may be continued for approximately 2 days to 1 week and then tapered and stopped.

Risperidone followed by conventional, high-potency antipsychotic agents such as haloperidol is currently preferred for the long-term management of psychotic symptoms that accompany dementia and agitation (Alexopoulos et al. 1998). However, olanzapine and quetiapine are gaining in popularity as first-line options. The use of all of the atypical antipsychotic agents at lower dosages offers a lower risk than conventional antipsychotic agents for causing EPS in long-term treatment of dementia. The use of antipsychotic agents is intended to decrease psychotic symptoms such as paranoia, delusions, hallucinations, and associated agitation and disruptive behaviors (e.g., screaming, combativeness, violence). Short- or long-term intervention with a antipsychotic agent must be specified in terms of describing target symptoms in order to select the optimal treatment and monitor the effect. Interventions for psychosis should be guided by the patient's level of distress and the risk to the patient and his or her caregivers. If there is little distress or danger, then reassurance and distraction may be all that is required. However, if a patient is distressed or exhibits significant agitation, combativeness, or violent behavior that puts others in danger, psychopharmacological intervention with a antipsychotic drug is clearly indicated. Similar guidelines apply for patients with milder forms of agitation or anxiety.

Many clinicians prefer antipsychotic drugs that fall between low- and high-potency profiles for conventional antipsychotics (e.g., perphenazine or loxapine); no data support the contention that these agents have fewer overall adverse effects. Thus, it is best to select an agent whose effects are less likely to cause problems for a given patient. For example, a high-potency agent such as haloperidol is best for a patient who is sensitive to anticholinergic agents. Similarly, a low-potency agent such as thioridazine may be best for a patient with parkinsonism or may more effectively benefit those with sundowning or sleep disturbances. Risperidone carries a lower risk of EPS at doses of 1–2 mg/day or less. Clozapine may be a good choice for patients with Parkinson's disease or Lewy body disease or others who cannot tolerate EPS. Likewise, quetiapine may be a good choice for a patient who needs sedation and is sensitive to EPS.

Suggested starting doses for risperidone are 0.25 mg twice daily with gradual increases of a maximum of 1.5–3 mg/day in divided doses or olanzapine initiated at a dose of 2.5 mg at bedtime and increased by increments of 2.5 mg to a maximum of 15 mg/day (Verma et al. 1998). For quetiapine, starting doses of 12.5–25 mg twice a day with an average of 50–400 mg is recommended.

The risk of more serious complications must be considered when weighing the potential benefits of antipsychotics in patients with dementia. The risk of TD may be as high as 30% and is greater with increased dose and longer duration of treatment; TD occurs more commonly in women and elderly persons in general (Jeste et al. 1995; Woemer et al. 1995). Another possible complication is neuroleptic malignant syndrome, which is rare but potentially lethal. Both of these complications have been reported with risperidone, but they occur at lower frequencies with atypical agents. Clozapine appears less likely to be associated with TD or neuroleptic malignant syndrome, but its use involves a significant risk of agranulocytosis, more common in elderly patients than in younger individuals (Salzman et al. 1995). Olanzapine and quetiapine have not been associated with either of these complications, but additional data and practice experience will characterize their effects in practice.

Antipsychotic agents are most commonly administered in the evening so that maximum blood levels occur while the patient is asleep and behavioral problems that peak in the evening hours (e.g., sundowning) are better improved. Because antipsychotic agents generally have longer half-lives, once-daily dosing is often sufficient; however, morning doses or twice-daily dosing may be helpful, depending on the patient's symptom pattern. On the whole, antipsychotic agents are given as standing doses rather than as-needed doses, but as-needed doses are appropriate for symptoms that occur infrequently. Oral administration is preferred, but intramuscular injection is sometimes used in an acute situation or if a patient is unable to take the medication by mouth. Very low doses of depot anti-psychotic medications (i.e., 1.25–3.75 mg per 2 weeks of fluphenazine dec-anoate) have been shown in a small open-label study to be effective in managing agitation in dementia (Gottlieb et al. 1988). Low starting doses are recommended (e.g., 0.5 mg/day of haloperidol, 10–25 mg/day of thi-oridazine, 2 mg/day of perphenazine, 1–2 mg/day of thiothixene, or 12.5 mg/day of clozapine). These dosages can be increased on the basis of re-sponse of target symptoms. The usual maximum daily dosages are 2–5 mg of haloperidol, 10–15 mg of thiothixene, 16–24 mg of perphenazine, 50–100 mg of thioridazine, 1–2 mg of risperidone, and 75–200 mg of clozapine, or equivalent dosages of other agents. Patients do best with doses below these maximums, but younger and less frail individuals may tolerate and respond to somewhat higher doses.

Given their side effects and potential toxicity, the risks and benefits of antipsychotic agents must be reassessed on an ongoing basis. The lowest effective dose should be sought, and emergent side effects should be first treated by dose reduction. The routine prescribing of anticholinergic agents should be avoided. In addition, periodic attempts to reduce or withdraw antipsychotic medications should be considered for all patients in the context of the probability of a relapse and the dangerousness of the target behaviors. Longer-term treatment of patients with agitation may re-quire several weeks of tapering after 1–6 months of treatment for mild ag-itation or 3–9 months of treatment for more severe forms of agitation (Alexopoulos et al. 1998). For patients with high medical comorbidity, an atypical antipsychotic agent such as risperidone or olanzapine is best.

Compared with conventional antipsychotic drugs, atypical antipsy-chotic agents promise improved side-effect profiles and better control of symptoms of agitation in dementia. Many patients receiving conventional antipsychotics could potentially benefit from a switch to an atypical anti-psychotic. Switching should occur in the context of persistent symptoma-tology, poor symptom control despite compliance, or persistent EPS (Weiden et al. 1997). From the caregiver's perspective, disruptiveness, burden, multiple crises, and setbacks are significant indicators of the po-tential benefit of switching. From the patient's perspective, degree of dis-tress from symptoms, secondary anxiety and depression, and impact on functional capacity are paramount.

Use of Antipsychotics in Long-term Care Facilities: Omnibus Reconciliation Act Guidelines

Antipsychotic agents are frequently prescribed for agitation in patients with dementia residing in long-term care facilities. Despite clinical practices and federal mandates that attempt to taper and stop these medications, empiric data regarding the cessation of treatment are limited. Bridges-Parlet et al. (1997) published a randomized, double-blind, baseline, controlled, 4-week trial with 36 institutionalized patients with AD. Of the 22 patients who were selected to be withdrawn from antipsychotics, 20 completed the 4-week, double-blind withdrawal. Of the 14 patients selected to continue antipsychotic agents, all completed the study. Generalizations of these results are limited. However, this study highlights the need for periodic assessment and withdrawal or tapering of drug.

Because of growing concerns about antipsychotics being overused, misused, or administered by individuals with little understanding of the risks and benefits, the United States Omnibus Reconciliation Act of 1987 (OBRA) guidelines were developed. OBRA guidelines describe the appropriate use of such medications (Beers et al. 1991; Semla et al. 1994). Since 1989, when the regulatory requirements were enacted, clinicians and long-term care facilities have been responsible for not overtreating dementia patients with antipsychotic medications (Health Care Financing Administration 1989). Rather than prescribe antipsychotics for vague indications that range from mild agitation to restlessness to fidgeting, clinicians are required to document the diagnostic indication for concurrent antipsychotic use (e.g., coexistent schizophrenia, psychosis, or acute delirium) (Sunderland 1996). Furthermore, the continued use of such medication must be justified in an ongoing way, even if the underlying diagnosis is considered appropriate (Table 12–4). As a result of these restrictions on antipsychotic agents, some studies have focused on the long-term effects of drug discontinuation in nursing homes rather than on drug initiation. For example, the OBRA regulations continue to have a significant impact on the prescribing patterns in nursing homes, in which approximately 22% of the residents still receive antipsychotic agents. Semla et al. (1994) have demonstrated that the dementia subset of nursing home populations is the one most likely to experience successful drug discontinuations. Patients resistant to changes in antipsychotic dosing are those with psychotic diagnoses or no evidence of dementia.

Table 12–4. Recognized indications for the use of antipsychotic agents in long-term care facilities

Appropriate indications
Acute psychotic episodes
Atypical psychosis
Brief reactive psychosis
Delusional disorder
Huntington's disease
Organic mental syndromes (including dementia and delirium) with associated psychotic and/or agitated behaviors[a]
Psychotic mood disorders (including mania & depression w/ psychotic features)
Schizoaffective disorder
Schizophrenia
Schizophreniform disorder
Short-term (<7 days) symptomatic treatment of hiccups, nausea, vomiting, or pruritus
Tourette's syndrome

Inappropriate indications[b]
Agitated behaviors that do not represent danger to the resident or others
Anxiety
Depression (without psychotic features)
Fidgeting
Impaired memory
Indifference to surroundings
Insomnia
Nervousness
Poor self care
Restlessness
Uncooperativeness
Unsociability
Wandering

Note. [a]Psychotic and agitated behaviors 1) have been quantitatively (no. of episodes) and objectively (e.g., biting, kicking, scratching) documented; 2) are not caused by preventable reasons; and 3) are causing the resident to present a danger to self or to others; *continuously* cry, scream, yell, or pace, if these specific behaviors cause an impairment in functional capacity, experience psychotic symptoms (e.g., hallucinations, paranoia, delusions) not exhibited as dangerous behaviors or crying, screaming, yelling, or pacing but that cause the resident distress or impairment in functional capacity.
[b]Antipsychotic agents should not be used if one or more of the indications listed is the only indication for use.
Source. Adapted from Health Care Financing Administration 1989.

References

Alexopoulos GS, Silver JM, Kahn DA, et al: Treatment of agitation in older persons with dementia, in Expert Consensus Guideline Series, Postgraduate Medical Specialist Report. Edited by Docherty JP, Frances A, Kahn DA. Minneapolis, MN, McGraw Hill, 1998, pp 21–42

Allen RL, Walker Z, D'Ath PJ, et al: Risperidone for psychotic and behavioral symptoms in Lewy body dementia. Lancet 346:185, 1995

Avorn J, Dreyer P, Connelly K, et al: Use of psychotropic medication and the quality of care in rest homes. N Engl J Med 320:227–232, 1989

Avorn J, Monane M, Everitt DE, et al: Clinical assessment of extrapyramidal signs in nursing home patients given antipsychotic medication. Arch Intern Med 154:1113–1117, 1994

Baldessarini RJ, Frankenburg FR: Clozapine: a novel antipsychotic agent. N Engl J Med 325:746–754, 1991

Barnes R, Veith R, Okimoto J, et al: Efficacy of antipsychotic medications in behaviorally disturbed dementia patients. Am J Psychiatry 139:1170–1174, 1982

Beers MH, Ouslander JG, Rollingher I, et al: Explicit criteria for determining inappropriate medication use in nursing home residents. Arch Intern Med 151:825–832, 1991

Bridges-Parlet S, Knopman D, Steffes S: Withdrawal of neuroleptic medications from institutionalized dementia patients: results of a double-blind, baseline-treatment-controlled pilot study. J Geriatr Psychiatry Neurol 10:119–126, 1997

Carlyle W, Ancill RJ, Sheldon L: Aggression in the demented patient: a double-blind study of loxapine versus haloperidol. Int Clin Psychopharmacol 8:103–108, 1993

Chacko R, Hurley R, Jankovic J: Clozapine use in diffuse Lewy body disease. J Neuropsychiatry Clin Neurosci 5:206–208, 1993

Clark WS, Street JS, Feldman PD, et al: The effects of olanzapine in reducing emergence of psychosis among nursing home patients with Alzheimer's disease. J Clin Psychiatry 62:34–40, 2001

Cohen-Mansfield J, Marx MS, Billig N, et al: A description of agitation in a nursing home. Gerontology 3:M77–M84, 1989

Cummings JL: Cholinesterase inhibitors: a new class of psychotropic compounds. Am J Psychiatry 157:4–15, 2000

Devanand DP, Levy SR: Neuroleptic treatment of agitation and psychosis in dementia. J Geriatr Psychiatry Neurol 8(suppl 1):18–27, 1995

Devanand DP, Brockington CD, Moody BJ, et al: Behavioral syndromes in Alzheimer's disease. International Psychogeriatrics 4:161–184, 1992

Devanand DP, Jacobs DM, Tang M, et al: The course of psychopathologic features in mild to moderate Alzheimer's disease. Arch Gen Psychiatry 54:257–263, 1997

Devanand DP, Marder K, Michaels KS, et al: A randomized, placebo-controlled dose-comparison trial of haloperidol for psychosis and disruptive behaviors in Alzheimer's disease. Am J Psychiatry 155:1512–1520, 1998

Deyn PP, Katz IR: Control of aggression and agitation in patients with dementia: efficacy and safety of risperidone. Int J Geriatr Psychiatry 15(suppl 1):514–522, 2000

Drevets WC, Rubin EH: Psychotic symptoms and the longitudinal course of dementia of the Alzheimer type. Biol Psychiatry 25:39–48, 1989

Emsley RA, Raniwalla J, Bailey PJ, et al: A comparison of the effects of quetiapine and haloperidol in schizophrenic patients with a history of demonstrated positive response to conventional antipsychotic treatment. Int Clin Psychopharmacol 61:185–189, 2000

Finkel SI, Lyons JS, Anderson RL, et al: A randomized, placebo-controlled trial of thiothixene in agitated, demented nursing home patients. Int J Geriatr Psychiatry 10:129–136, 1995

Gerlach J, Peacock L: New antipsychotics: the present status. Int Clin Psychopharmacol 10(suppl 3):39–48, 1995

Goldberg RJ, Goldberg J: Risperidone for dementia-related disturbed behavior in nursing home residents: a clinical experience. International Psychogeriatrics 9:65–68, 1997

Gottlieb G, McAllister T, Gur R: Depot neuroleptics in the treatment of behavioral disorders in patients with Alzheimer's disease. J Am Geriatr Soc 36:619–621, 1988

Graham SR, Kokkinidis L: Clozapine inhibits limbic system kindling: implications for antipsychotic action. Brain Res Bull 30:597–605, 1993

Haller E, Binder RL, McNeil DE: Violence in geriatric patients with dementia. Bull Am Acad Psychiatry Law 17:183–188, 1989

Health Care Financing Administration. Medicare and Medicaid: requirements for long-term care facilities: final rule with request for comments. Federal Register 54:5316–5373, 1989

Herrmann N, Lanctot KL: From transmitters to treatment: the pharmacotherapy of behavioural disturbances in dementia. Can J Psychiatry 42(suppl 1):51–64, 1997

Herrmann N, Rivard MF, Flynn M, et al: Risperidone for the treatment of behavioral disturbances in dementia: a case series. J Neuropsychiatry Clin Neurosci 10:220–223, 1998

Jeste DV, Lacro JP, Gilbert PL, et al: Treatment of late-life schizophrenia with neuroleptics. Schizophr Bull 19:817–830, 1993

Jeste DV, Caliguiri MP, Paulsen JS, et al: Risk of tardive dyskinesia in older patients: a prospective longitudinal study of 266 outpatients. Arch Gen Psychiatry 52:756–765, 1995

Katz IR, Jeste DV, Mintzer JE, et al: Comparison of risperidone and placebo for psychosis and behavioral disturbances associated with dementia: a randomized, double-blind trial. Risperidone Study Group. J Clin Psychiatry 60:107–115, 1999

Keltner NL, Folks DG: Psychopharmacology for elderly patients, in Handbook of Psychotropic Drugs, 2nd Edition. St. Louis, MO, CV Mosby, 1997, pp 391–421

Lee H, Cooney JM, Lawlor BA: Case report: the use of risperidone, an atypical neuroleptic, in Lewy body disease. Int J Geriatr Psychiatry 9:415–417, 1994

Madhusoodanan S, Brenner R, Araujo L, et al: Efficacy of risperidone treatment for psychoses associated with schizophrenia, schizoaffective disorder, bipolar disorder, or senile dementia in 11 geriatric patients: a case series. J Clin Psychiatry 56:514–518, 1995

Meco G, Alessandria A, Bonifati V, et al: Risperidone for treating dementia-associated aggression (letter). Am J Psychiatry 152:1239, 1994

Meltzer HY: Clinical studies on the mechanism of action of clozapine: the dopamine serotonin hypothesis of schizophrenia. Psychopharmacology 99:188–197, 1989

Meltzer HY: The mechanism of action of novel antipsychotic drugs. Schizophr Bull 17:263–287, 1991

Nacasch N, Dolberg O, Hirschmann S, et al: Clozapine for the treatment of agitated-depressed patients with cognitive impairment: a report of three cases. Clin Neuropharmacol 21:132–134, 1998

Oberholzer AF, Hendricksen C, Monsch AU, et al: Safety and effectiveness of low-dose clozapine in psychogeriatric patients: a preliminary study. International Psychogeriatrics 4:187–195, 1992

Petrie WM, Ban TA, Berney S, et al: Loxapine in psychogeriatrics: a placebo and standard controlled clinical investigation. J Clin Psychopharmacol 2:122–126, 1982

Rabins PV, Mace NL, Lucas MJ: The impact of dementia on the family. JAMA 248:333–335, 1982

Rada RT, Kellner R: Thiothixene in the treatment of geriatric patients with chronic organic brain syndrome. J Am Geriatr Soc 24:105–107, 1976

Raskind M, Risse S, Lampe T: Dementia and antipsychotic drugs. J Clin Psychiatry 48:16–18, 1987

Raskind MA, Sadowsky CH, Sigmund WR, et al: Effect of tacrine on language, praxis, and noncognitive behavioral problems in Alzheimer's disease. Arch Neurol 54:836–840, 1997

Reisberg B, Borenstein J, Salob SP, et al: Behavioral symptoms in Alzheimer's disease: phenomenology and treatment. J Clin Psychiatry 48:9–15, 1987

Reisberg B, Franssen E, Sclan SG, et al: Stage-specific incidence of potentially remediable behavioral symptoms in aging and Alzheimer's disease: a study of 120 patients using the BEHAVE-AD. Bull Clin Neurosci 54:95–112, 1989

Rosen J, Zubenko GS: Emergence of psychosis and depression in the longitudinal evaluation of Alzheimer's disease. Biol Psychiatry 29:224–232, 1991

Rubin EH, Morris JC, Berg L: The progression of personality changes in senile dementia of the Alzheimer's type. J Am Geriatr Soc 35:721–725, 1987

Salzman C, Vaccaro B, Lieff J, et al: Clozapine in older patients with psychosis and behavioral disruption. Am J Geriatr Psychiatry 3:26–33, 1995

Schneider LS, Pollock VE, Lyness SA: A meta-analysis of controlled trials of neuroleptic treatment in dementia. J Am Geriatr Soc 38:553–563, 1990

Semla TP, Palla K, Poddig B, et al: Effect of the Omnibus Reconciliation Act of 1987 on antipsychotic prescribing in nursing home residents. J Am Geriatr Soc 42:648–652, 1994

Small GW, Jarvik LF: The dementia syndrome. Lancet 11:1443–1445, 1982

Stern Y, Mayeux R, Sano M, et al: Predictors of disease course in patients with probable Alzheimer's disease. Neurology 37:1649–1653, 1987

Street JS, Clark WS, Gannon KS, et al: Olanzapine treatment of psychotic and behavioral symptoms in patients with Alzheimer disease in nursing care facilities: a double-blind, randomized, placebo-controlled trial. Arch Gen Psychiatry 57:968–976, 2000

Sunderland T: Treatment of the elderly suffering from psychosis and dementia. J Clin Psychiatry 57(suppl 9):53–56, 1996

Swearer JM, Drachman DA, O'Donnell BF, et al: Troublesome and disruptive behaviors in dementia. J Am Geriatr Soc 36:784–790, 1988

Tariot PN: Treatment strategies for agitation and psychosis in dementia. J Clin Psychiatry 57(suppl 14):21–29, 1996

Tune L, Carr S, Hoag E, et al: Anticholinergic effects of drugs commonly prescribed for the elderly: potential means for assessing risk of delirium. Am J Psychiatry 149:1393–1394, 1992

Verma SD, Davidoff DA, Kambhampati KK: Management of the agitated elderly patient in the nursing home: the role of the atypical antipsychotics. J Clin Psychiatry 59(suppl 19):50–55, 1998

Weiden PG, Aquila R, Dalheim L, et al: Switching antipsychotic medications. J Clin Psychiatry 58(suppl 10):63–72, 1997

Woemer MG, Alvir JMJ, Kane JM, et al: Neuroleptic treatment of elderly patients. Psychopharmacol Bull 31:333–337, 1995

Workman RH Jr, Orengo CA, Bakey AA, et al: The use of risperidone for psychosis and agitation in demented patients with Parkinson's disease. J Neuropsychiatry Clin Neurosci 9:594–597, 1997

Wragg RE, Jeste DV: Overview of depression and psychosis in Alzheimer's disease. Am J Psychiatry 146:577–587, 1989

Zarate CA Jr, Baldessarini RJ, Siegel AJ, et al: Risperidone in the elderly: a pharmacoepidemiologic study. J Clin Psychiatry 58:311–317, 1997

CHAPTER 13

Beta-Blockers, Benzodiazepines, and Other Miscellaneous Agents

Kari L. Franson, Pharm.D.
Deanna Chesley, Pharm.D.
John S. Kennedy, M.D., F.R.C.P.C.

Since the development of the Omnibus Reconciliation Act of 1987 (OBRA), clinicians have been searching for alternative pharmacotherapy for the behavioral disturbances associated with dementia. However, reviews of the literature before this legislation—and since the legislation has been enforced—provide little information for the proper use of alternative agents for agitation (American Psychiatric Association 1996). There has been a lack of well-designed studies in clearly defined populations to assess the usefulness of these agents. Case reports, open-label trials, and clinical lore continue to drive clinicians to use these agents when other interventions fail. A review of the literature seems to suggest that because the pathophysiology of dementia is multifactorial, any centrally acting agent might have an impact on the disease. In this chapter we review the psychotherapeutic agents that have a significant body of literature that do not fall into other larger categories. In this chapter we review the significant body of literature regarding the use of beta-blockers, benzodiazepines, and other miscellaneous agents for the treatment of mild behavioral disturbances associated with dementia.

Beta-blockers

Beta-blockers have been used in the realm of neuropsychiatry for more than 20 years. Clinical indications for their use has included anxiety disorders; attention-deficit disorder; personality disorders; schizophrenia; akathisia; and agitated or aggressive behaviors associated with dementias, seizure disorders, metabolic disorders, head injuries, and developmental disorders (Haspel 1995; Volavka 1988). Theoretical benefits of beta-blockers include fewer side effects and little effect on cognitive performance (Ratey and Gordon 1994); however, the clinical role for the use in agitated behaviors of the various beta-blockers is not well documented.

The neurochemical basis for agitation and aggression is unclear, but a hyper-adrenergic state is one hypothesis. Four findings support this hypothesis: 1) norepinephrine has been found to amplify aggression in animal models; 2) the alpha-2 antagonist yohimbine, an agent that inhibits the negative feedback blockade of norepinephrine, has also been used to induce anxiety and agitation in laboratory animals; 3) protriptyline, a tricyclic agent that blocks the reuptake of norepinephrine, enhanced rage in treated felines; and 4) the proposed mechanism of action for beta-blocker use in agitation is the inhibition of sympathetic outflow from the central nervous system (CNS). Several rat and human studies have demonstrated that beta-blockers inhibit aggressive behavior (Smith and Perry 1992; Weiler et al. 1988).

In a recent review of beta-blocker use for agitation, Schneider and Sobin (1991) found response rates to be more than 80% in open prospective studies of mixed organic samples. This compares with just 67% in double-blind studies, with no studies comparing the treated patients with subjects receiving placebo. Unfortunately, use in dementia patients was unclear. The dosages used ranged from 60 to 520 mg/day of propranolol to 40 to 60 mg/day of pindolol. The target symptoms that were most responsive included impulsivity, hostility, and assaultiveness. Most adverse experiences were related to either the cardiovascular system or the CNS. Yudofsky (1987) described a 12-step guide for the appropriate clinical use of propranolol in psychiatry.

Pharmacokinetics and Pharmacodynamics

Originally it was believed that beta-blockers had to be used centrally to block the adrenergic receptors; however, the use of more hydrophilic agents such as naldolol suggests that crossing the blood–brain barrier is not required for efficacy (Ratey et al. 1992). The partial beta-adrenergic agonist-antagonist pindolol has also been used with some degree of success (Greendyke and Kanter 1986).

Side Effects

Beta-blockers have been reported to cause hypotension, bradycardia, orthostasis, dizziness, impotence, depression, sedation, and bronchospasm. After 2 weeks of therapy, these agents should be tapered slowly to avoid tachycardia from adrenergic rebound.

It has been previously stated that the clinical usefulness and particular patient populations in which beta-blockers would be beneficial has not been established. The one possible caveat to that statement is use of beta-blockers for patients with agitation or aggression secondary to akathisia. Several studies have found propranolol to be helpful for akathisia and normally well tolerated (Adler et al. 1987; Kramer et al. 1988). In conclusion, the use of beta-blockers is not well substantiated. Most clinicians continue to use these agents to "take the edge off" and normally use them in combination with other agents. Hypotension and rebound tachycardia should be monitored carefully because of the sensitivity of the geriatric population to these adverse effects.

Benzodiazepines

Benzodiazepines may be effective in treating patients with agitation by providing sedation, muscle relaxation, and antianxiety actions (Ancil 1991; Coccaro 1990). However, benzodiazepines are also associated with many adverse effects, especially in the elderly (Cummings et al. 1991; Goldney 1977; Gudex 1991). To prevent overuse of these drugs and associated adverse outcomes, the OBRA established guidelines for the appropriate indication, dosage, and duration of psychotropic drug therapy, including benzodiazepines (Borson and Doane 1997). Although there may be a role for these drugs in the treatment of acute agitation, there is no evidence that long-term therapy is beneficial when taking into account both the control of behavior and drug side effects.

Benzodiazepines appear to exert their effects by enhancing γ-aminobutyric acid (GABA) response. The drugs are thought to interact in a macromolecular complex that includes GABA receptors, benzodiazepine receptors, and chloride channels. The interaction causes an opening of the chloride channels, which ultimately results in sedation, decreased anxiety, muscle relaxation, and antiseizure activity. There appear to be at least three types of benzodiazepine receptors (types 1, 2, and 3), with most benzodiazepines being nonselective to the subtypes. Although the exact clinical significance of the three receptor types is unknown, the hypnotic zolpidem (Ambien) appears to only interact with the type 1 receptor, which may help to explain the decreased incidence of side effects associated with zolpidem compared with the benzodiazepines.

The benzodiazepines differ in terms of their pharmacokinetic profiles. In general, elderly patients are more efficient at eliminating drugs that are not oxidized. Therefore, based on half-life, absence of active metabolites, and lack of oxidation, lorazepam, oxazepam, and temazepam are potentially the safest drugs to use in the elderly.

Side Effects

Benzodiazepines are associated with significant side effects in elderly patients, including increased agitation and disinhibition. Chronically, they may also lead to dependency, increased risk of falls and hip fractures, cognitive impairment, and confusion (Cummings et al. 1991; Gudex 1991; Lechin 1996). Benzodiazepines decrease rapid eye movement (REM) sleep and stage 3 and 4 sleep. The full impact of these changes is unknown (Lechin et al. 1996).

Significant Drug–Drug Interactions

In general, any drug that depresses the CNS may potentiate the effects of benzodiazepines. Several cytochrome P450–mediated interactions should also be noted. The most significant include interaction with inhibitors of the 3A4 isoenzyme, including nefazodone, cisapride, astemizole, macrolides, and possibly grapefruit juice. All of these inhibitors may increase sensitivity to the benzodiazepines. Smoking may cause the induction of enzymes that metabolize the benzodiazepines and result in decreased sensitivity to the benzodiazepine (Michalets 1998).

Sedating Antihistamines

Drugs that fall into the class of antihistamines are often used to curb agitation and combative behaviors in psychiatric patients. According to theory, anticholinergic agents should inhibit the aggressiveness induced by cholinergic stimulation in the hypothalamus. However, only a few old studies support this theory, and clinical experience suggests that the opposite is true. Patients with dementia have decreasing cholinergic activity throughout the duration of the disease, yet they are increasingly combative or agitated. Much of the calming effects of the anticholinergic agents can be attributed to the inhibition of histamine-1 receptors. Unfortunately, patients quickly become tolerant to the sedative properties of histaminergic blockade.

Despite this, anticholinergic agents such as diphenhydramine and hydroxyzine are often used for sedation in younger patients. These anticholinergics are equipotent and are typically dosed at 25–50 mg. However, because of the strong anticholinergic effects of these agents, routine use in the elderly is not warranted. Problems with hypotension, tachycardia, blurred vision, urinary retention, and confusion limit the usefulness of anticholinergic drugs in the elderly population.

Cholinergic Agents

Many of the new therapies aimed at improving cognitive function are now being investigated for their potential for improving behavioral disturbances in patients with dementia. For example, behavioral agitation has been seen in patients without dementia who are receiving anticholinergic agents. Patients given physostigmine (an acetylcholinesterase inhibitor [ACHEI]) demonstrated reduced agitation (Milam and Bennett 1987). Studies are now investigating whether the same effect occurs in patients with Alzheimer's disease (AD) who are deficient in acetylcholine. The agents being given are cholinesterase inhibitors, which work by binding to acetyl and butryl cholinesterases. This inhibition blocks the breakdown of acetylcholine, thereby elevating the amount of acetylcholine in the synapse.

Literature Review

Tacrine, donepezil, rivastigmine, and other ACHEIs have been shown to improve behaviors in several studies (Kaufer 1996; Morris et al. 1998). To evaluate patients' responses to therapy, researchers have been using scales such as the Alzheimer's Disease Assessment Scale—noncognitive (ADAS-noncog; Rosen et al. 1984) and the Neuropsychiatric Inventory (NPI; Cummings et al. 1994).

Unfortunately, in the earlier studies with tacrine, most of the focus was on cognitive enhancement; therefore, these studies' authors have mentioned improvement in behavioral aspects without providing distinct data (Knapp et al. 1994). Later studies using donepezil (5 or 10 mg/day) or rivastigmine (1–4 or 6–12 mg/day) versus placebo did show improvement on CIBIC-Plus scores after 26 weeks of study (Corey-Bloom et al. 1998; Rogers et al. 1998). Again, these data are difficult to interpret because the studies focused on cognitive factors and because patients with significant behavioral problems were excluded or treated with other therapies. Perhaps the best data presented have been with metrifonate. In one study, the investigators found that patients receiving metrifonate were less likely to develop behavioral symptoms such as agitation, hallucinations, and delusions on the NPI scale than patients taking placebo (Morris et al. 1998). Further development with metrifonate has since stopped because of side effects, but the design of this trial is now being replicated using other ACHEIs. It is unfortunate that there have been no head-to-head trials of these cholinergic agents with other behavioral therapy interventions.

Doses

The only cholinergic drugs currently available in the United States for use in patients with dementia are tacrine, donepezil, rivastigmine, and galantamine. Behavioral improvements have been studied at dosages that also improve cognitive functioning. Therefore, it is recommended to dose these drugs according to guidelines. Donepezil should be started at 5 mg/day and increased to 10 mg/day if clinically necessary. Rivastigmine is started at 1.5 mg twice daily and increased to 6 mg twice daily as tolerated. Tacrine should be started at 10 mg four times daily and increased by 40 mg/day (10 mg per dose) every 6 weeks. Best results have been seen at 30 or 40 mg four times daily.

Side Effects

As a class, the most common side effects include nausea, diarrhea, abdominal upset, dizziness, myalgia, and headache. With all these agents, the gastrointestinal side effects are dose related, and rapid increases to high doses are associated with worsening symptoms. Because of the acridine structure of tacrine, there is also a risk of hepatotoxicity. Therefore, clinicians need to monitor liver enzyme levels every *other* week for the first 18 weeks.

Significant Drug–Drug Interactions

Tacrine is metabolized by the cytochrome P450 1A2 isoenzyme. Therefore, inhibitors of 1A2 increase serum concentrations of tacrine, and inducers (e.g., cigarette smoking) decrease the concentrations. Rivastigmine is unique among the ACHEIs because it has no significant potential for P450-based pharmacokinetic drug–drug interactions.

Selegiline

Selegiline is a monoamine oxidase inhibitor (MAOI) with relative selectivity for MAO type B at low doses (<11 mg/day) (Gelman et al. 1998). Monoamine oxidase (MAO) is an enzyme that is responsible for the degradation of dopamine, norepinephrine, and serotonin. MAO type B is found primarily in the central nervous system and type A in the peripheral. Inhibition of MAO type A is associated with cardiovascular-related side effects such as hypotension and interactions such as hypertensive crisis with the coadministration of sympathomimetics. Selegiline may also possess dopaminergic effects apart from its interaction with MAO (Gelman et al. 1997). Patients with dementia have been found to exhibit structural and functional disturbances of catecholamine and indoleamine systems, including increased levels of MAO. Thus, selegiline may help to restore normal neurotransmitter functioning, which could lead to improvement in behavior, cognition, and mood (Schneider and Sobin 1991; Tariot et al. 1987). Selegiline also has antioxidant effects that could aid in the prevention of neuronal damage. A recent study (Sano et al. 1997) demonstrated that the administration of selegiline in patients with moderately severe AD may delay the occurrence of death, institutionalization, loss of the ability to perform basic activities of daily living, or severe dementia.

Literature Review

A few small studies have demonstrated improvement in behavior that could be attributed to selegiline. Tariot et al. (1987) administered low-dose (10 mg/day) and high-dose (40 mg/day) selegiline to 17 patients with dementia in a double-blind serial treatment. Behavioral changes were periodically assessed via the Brief Psychiatric Rating Scale (BPRS), qualitative observation, and global impression of change. The mean total BPRS decreased during the 10-mg/day therapy, primarily because of decreases in the factors of anxiety or depression and activation. Qualitative behavioral observations showed a clinically significant decrease in tension, retardation, and depressive ideation, more during the 10-mg/day therapy. However, global clinical impression results demonstrated no significant change in any of the patients. Transient increases in irritability were noted in half of the patients, primarily during the therapy with 40 mg/day. Other side effects were also more significant during the 40-mg/day therapy and included orthostasis, apraxia, bradykinesia, and influenza-like syndrome after rapid drug withdrawal.

Goad et al. (1991) studied the effects of selegiline in eight patients with AD. Selegiline 10 mg/day was administered for 8 weeks, and behavior changes were assessed by the patients' caregivers via the Behavioral Path ology in Alzheimer's Disease Rating Scale (BEHAVE-AD) and the Caregiver Burden Scale. Of the eight patients, three dropped out—one because of increased aggressive behavior, one because of increased agitation and hallucinations, and one for personal reasons. Two of the remaining five patients required a lowering of the dosage to 5 mg/day because of side effects. Results showed no significant change in behavior from baseline in terms of both the BEHAVE-AD and Caregiver Burden Scale. However, according to the authors, there was a clinically significant improvement in the behavior symptoms of paranoid and delusional ideation, hallucinations, activity disturbances, anxiety, and phobias.

Lastly, Schneider et al. (1991) administered 5 mg of selegiline twice a day to 14 patients in an open-label pilot study. Behavior was assessed via the BPRS, Cornell Scale for Depression, and Relatives Assessment of Global Symptomatology (RAGS-E). There was one dropout secondary to agitation and insomnia, but no other side effects occurred. A significant decrease in the factors of depression and agitation of the BPRS was noted. There was also a significant decrease in sadness, irritability, and agitation on the Cornell scale and a significant decrease in the RAGS-E rating pre- versus post-therapy.

Doses

The optimal dosage of selegiline is 10 mg/day (Gelman et al. 1997; Tariot 1987). At higher doses, selectivity for MAO type B is lost and the inhibition of MAO type A becomes more significant, along with the associated side effects. Furthermore, therapeutic benefits of the drug are not significantly increased at higher doses.

Side Effects

The most common side effects include nausea, dizziness, lightheadedness, fainting, and abdominal pain (Gelman et al. 1997).

Significant Drug–Drug Interactions

Eldepryl has been associated with symptoms such as stupor, muscular rigidity, severe agitation, autonomic instability, and elevated temperature when coadministered with meperidine, tricyclic antidepressants, serotonin reuptake inhibitors, and nonselective MAOIs (Gelman et al. 1997). Therefore, it is recommended to wait 14 days after discontinuing Eldepryl before adding these medications. If a patient has been receiving fluoxetine, it is recommended that he or she wait 5 weeks before adding Eldepryl (Gelman et al. 1997).

References

Adler L, Angrist B, Peselow E, et al: Noradrenergic mechanisms in akathisia: treatment with propranolol and clonidine. Psychopharmacol Bull 149:42–45, 1987

American Psychiatric Association: Practice guidelines for the treatment of patients with Alzheimer's disease and other dementias of late life. Am J Psychiatry 154:1–39, 1996

Ancil R, Carlyle R, Liang R, et al: Agitation in the demented elderly: a role for benzodiazepines? Int Clin Psychopharmacol 6:141–146, 1991

Borson S, Doane K: The impact of OBRA-87 on psychotropic drug prescribing in skilled nursing facilities. Psychiatr Serv 48:1289–1296, 1997

Coccaro E, Kramer E, Zemishlany Z, et al: Pharmacologic treatment of non-cognitive behavioral disturbances in elderly demented patients. Am J Psychiatry 147:1640–1645, 1990

Corey-Bloom J, Anand R, Veach J: A randomized trial evaluating the efficacy and safety of ENA 713 (rivastigmine tartrate), a new acetylcholinesterase inhibitor, in patients with mild to moderately severe Alzheimer's disease. Int J Geriatr Psychiatry 1:55–65, 1998

Cummings JL, Mega M, Gray K, et al: The Neuropsychiatric Inventory: comprehensive assessment of psychopathology in dementia. Neurology 44:2308–2314, 1994

Cummings R, Miller P, Kelsey J, et al: Medications and multiple falls in elderly people: the St. Louis OASIS study. Age and Aging 20:455–461, 1991

Gelman CR, Rumack BH, Hutchinson TA (eds): DRUGDEX System. Englewood, CO, Micromedex, Inc, 1997

Goad D, Davis C, Liem P, et al: The use of selegiline in Alzheimer's patients with behavior problems. J Clin Psychiatry 52:342–345, 1991

Goldney R: Paradoxical reaction to a new minor tranquilizers. Med J Aust 1:139–140, 1977

Greendyke RM, Kanter DR: Therapeutic effects of pindolol on behavioral disturbances associated with organic brain disease: a double blind study. J Clin Psychiatry 47:423–426, 1986

Gudex C: Adverse effects of benzodiazepines. Soc Sci Med 33:587–596, 1991

Haspel T: Beta-blockers and the treatment of aggression. Harv Rev Psychiatry 2:274–281, 1995

Kaufer DI, Cummings JL, Christine D: Effect of tacrine on behavioral symptoms in Alzheimer's disease: an open study. J Geriatr Psychiatry Neurol 9:1–6, 1996

Knapp MJ, Knopman DS, Soloman PR, et al: A 30-week randomized controlled trial of high dose tacrine in patients with Alzheimer's disease. JAMA 271:985–991, 1994

Kramer MS, Gorkin RA, Di Johnson C, et al: Propranolol in the treatment of neuroleptic-induced akathisia (NIA) in schizophrenics: a double-blind, placebo-controlled study. Biol Psychiatry 24:823–827, 1988

Lechin F, van der Dijs, Benaim M: Benzodiazepines: Tolerability in elderly patients. Psychother Psychosom 65:171–182, 1996

Michalets E: Update: Clinically significant cytochrome P-450 drug interactions. Pharmacotherapy 18:84–112, 1998

Milam SB, Bennett CR: Physostigmine reversal of drug induced paradoxical excitement. Int J Oral Maxillofac Surg 16:190–193, 1987

Morris JC, Cyrus PA, Orazem J, et al: Metrifonate benefits cognitive, behavioral and global function in patients with Alzheimer's disease. Neurology 50:1222–1230, 1998

Ratey JJ, Gordon A: The psychopharmacology of aggression: toward a new day. Psychopharmacol Bull 29:65–73, 1994

Ratey JJ, Sorgi P, O'Driscoll GA, et al: Nadolol to treat aggressive and psychiatric symptomatology in chronic psychiatric inpatients: a double-blind, placebo-controlled study. J Clin Psychiatry 53:41–46, 1992

Rogers SL, Farlow MR, Doody RS, et al: A 24 week double blind placebo controlled trial of donepezil in patients with Alzheimer's disease. Neurology 50:136–145, 1998

Rosen WG, Mohs RC, Davis KL: A new rating scale for Alzheimer's disease. Am J Psychiatry 141:1356–1364, 1984

Sano M, Ernesto C, Thomas R, et al: A controlled trial of selegiline, alpha-tocopherol, or both as treatment for Alzheimer's disease. N Engl J Med 336:1216–1222, 1997

Schneider LS, Sobin PB: Non-neuroleptic medications in the management of agitation in Alzheimer's disease and other dementia: a selective review. Int J Geriatr Psychiatry 6:691–708, 1991

Schneider L, Pollock V, Zemansky M, et al: A pilot study of low-dose L-deprenyl in Alzheimer's disease. J Geriatr Psychiatry Neurol 4:143–148, 1991

Smith D, Perry PJ: Non-neuroleptic treatment of disruptive behaviors in organic mental syndrome. Ann Pharmacother 26:1400–1408, 1992

Tariot P, Cohen R, Sunderland T, et al: L-Deprenyl in Alzheimer's disease. Arch Gen Psychiatry 44:427–433, 1987

Volavka J: Can aggressive behavior in humans be modified by beta blockers? Postgrad Med 29:163–168, 1988

Weiler PG, Mungas D, Bernick C: Propranolol for the control of disruptive behavior in senile dementia. J Geriatr Psychiatry Neurol 1:226–230, 1988

Yudofsky S: 12-step guide to the clinical use of propranolol. Psychiatr Ann 17:6, 1987

CHAPTER 14

Electroconvulsive Therapy

Elizabeth Cookson, M.D.
Donald P. Hay, M.D.

Verbal and physical agitation strongly predict functional decline and out-of-home placement for patients with dementia. Agitated behavior often reflects a patient's distress and can also be extremely distressing and disruptive for caregivers and families. Practitioners and researchers have investigated multiple therapies for the management of this difficult clinical problem, and previous chapters have discussed the indications, efficacy, and risks of these drug and nondrug interventions. However, what can be done if the patient does not tolerate or respond to these therapies? Additional treatment strategies are needed. In this chapter we discuss the use of electroconvulsive therapy (ECT) for agitated patients with dementia, particularly when agitation is secondary to depression.

Development of pharmacotherapeutic and psychotherapeutic interventions for dementia has outpaced ECT research and clinical practice, possibly because of the often-politicized nature of this treatment modality. In the public's perception, ECT is frequently thought of as an extraordinary treatment and believed to be overly intrusive, outdated, and/or traumatic. Even among some psychiatrists, ECT is often seen as a treatment of last resort. Yet ECT may be the treatment of choice if rapid relief of symptoms is necessary, such as with starvation or severe suicidality; if medications are contraindicated because of side effects or drug–drug interactions; if the patient has been successfully treated with ECT during past episodes of illness; or if the patient's illness has been refractory to all medication attempts.

Well-established indications for ECT include major depressive disorder, depression secondary to a general medical condition (identified as "organic affective disorder" in DSM-III [American Psychiatric Association 1980] and DSM-III-R [American Psychiatric Association 1987]), mania, and some psychotic disorders (Abrams 1997; American Psychiatric Association 1990, 2001). These conditions frequently culminate in agitation in patients with dementia. Coexisting depression may contribute to the cognitive decline of these patients. For depressed patients, ECT offers more rapid symptom relief; for delusional patients, ECT may reduce the use of antipsychotic medications, with side effects such as anticholinergic toxicity, orthostasis, extrapyramidal symptoms, and tardive dyskinesia. Vigorous treatment of comorbid psychiatric disorders can lead to significant improvement in the quality of life for patients with dementia. ECT may have an important role for select patients.

ECT and Dementia

With modern ECT practice, there are no absolute contraindications. ECT can be safely administered to most patients with neurological disease, including those with dementia (Zwil and Pelchat 1994). Given ECT's efficacy in depression and the frequent co-occurrence of depression and dementia, a considerable literature on ECT for patients with dementia might be expected to exist; however, the data available on safety and efficacy are limited to case studies.

Price and McAllister (1989) reviewed 26 articles reporting on 43 patients with dementia and depression treated with ECT. Thirteen of 19 patients (68%) with Alzheimer's disease showed a positive response to ECT; 11 of the patients treated (58%) showed no worsening of cognitive or memory symptoms, and 6 of these (32% of the larger group) actually showed an improvement in cognitive functioning. All six patients with worsened cognitive function cleared with time, although it took 65 days for one patient. Only one of eight patients with depression, dementia, and Parkinson's disease showed a transient (4- to 6-week) worsening of intellectual function, although the antidepressant response in this group was not impressive. The five patients with depression, dementia, and Huntington's disease all had positive responses without cognitive side effects. ECT offered significant improvement in depressive symptoms for the six patients with multi-infarct dementia; 50% of this group showed cognitive or memory improvement. (The type of ECT was frequently not specified; bilateral ECT was more often associated with significant memory impairment.)

Nelson and Rosenberg (1991) described the use of ECT in 21 patients with dementia. The diagnoses treated were major depression, dysthymia, and organic affective disorder. Twelve patients had failed adequate drug trials, four had medical contraindications to pharmacotherapy, two were refusing to eat or drink, and four had responded well to ECT in the past. All patients were initially treated with nondominant unilateral stimuli. In this naturalistic series, there was no significant difference in response to ECT between the patients in the dementia group and 84 nondemented depressed patients treated with ECT, although the women with dementia had less relief of depression than those in the control group. Post-ECT confusion correlated with the patient's degree of dementia, was not a cause of treatment interruption, and did not affect ECT's efficacy against depression. Although those in the group with dementia were somewhat older, they had no more cardiac complications than the control group.

Schnur et al. (1989) described the treatment of five patients with aggression and organic delusional disorder. In this small series, aggression decreased for all patients with little effect on their psychoses. Seizures decreased in the four patients with treatment-resistant seizure disorders. The investigators hypothesized that the anticonvulsant effect of ECT may contribute to an antiaggressive effect.

Electroconvulsive therapy has also been suggested for treatment of agitated patients with dementia (Hay et al. 1995). Carlyle et al. (1991) described the administration of bilateral ECT to three patients with dementia after multiple medication trials failed to relieve verbal agitation (described as "needless, unstimulated screaming, yelling, moaning"). Two of the three patients had no clear history of a past or present major depressive episode. Screaming stopped early in each ECT course. Holmberg et al. (1996) reported the case of an elderly woman with vascular dementia and severe agitation. ECT was used after pharmacological and nonpharmacological interventions failed, and the patient showed dramatic improvement. Her behavioral symptoms returned when maintenance treatments were delayed.

In the next four sections, we briefly review ECT technique, with a focus on issues specific to patients with dementia. Several excellent texts are available for more detailed discussions of this therapy (e.g., Abrams 1997; Coffey 1993).

ECT Work-Up

Before beginning ECT, a thorough diagnostic assessment should be completed to eliminate medical diagnoses, including pain complaints that could explain the patient's behavioral or affective symptoms (see Chapter 6). In this patient group, brain imaging (by either computed tomography or magnetic resonance imaging) may be helpful to screen for abnormal vasculature, characterize possible white matter lesions or atrophy, and evaluate for conditions (e.g., a space-occupying lesion) associated with increased intracranial pressure. (ECT can be given safely and effectively to patients with many central nervous system abnormalities, but conditions involving increased intracranial pressure or recent hemorrhage substantially increase the risks.) Baseline cognitive testing is very helpful in following postictal and interictal confusion (see discussion below).

Pretreatment medical assessment and management should focus special attention on the problems of elderly patients, including cardiac and pulmonary status, musculoskeletal problems, and the potential for gastroesophageal reflux. Essential to efficacious treatment is an adequate seizure; therefore, drugs that raise the seizure threshold, such as anticonvulsant agents, should be tapered or stopped when possible. Medications that increase seizure duration, such as theophylline and lidocaine, should also be avoided. Careful evaluation of the patient's teeth, dentures, and dental work is important, given the high number of weakened dental structures that may be subject to fracture or breakage during the stimulus or subsequent seizure. Acute closed-angle glaucoma or a retinal detachment should be evaluated carefully and stabilized before starting the course of ECT and may require close management by an ophthalmologist during the treatment series.

Informed Consent

There are three components to the consent process (American Psychiatric Association 1990). First, adequate information must be provided. Education of the patient and his or her family is a critical part of a successful course of ECT. Descriptive pamphlets and videos that explain the technique, allay fears, reduce misconceptions, and answer questions are helpful adjuncts to face-to-face instruction. A pre-ECT conference that includes all interested parties should review the patient's diagnosis, the nature of the proposed therapy, the treatment alternatives, and the risks and benefits of each choice. Target symptoms should be clearly delineated, with the anticipated time to their remission. For patients with dementia and depression, a strong family history of depression may exist, including past family experiences with ECT. Outcomes of past ECT treatments received by the patient or family members should be explored.

The second component entails "a patient who is capable of understanding and acting intelligently upon such information" (American Psychiatric Association 1990, p. 64). ECT presents intrinsic challenges to the consent process because of the repeated administration of treatments and the possible occurrence of memory disruption during the course of treatments (see discussion below). Caregivers should expect to regularly reevaluate the patient's mental status and to periodically revisit the consent process. When recommending ECT for the treatment of a patient with dementia, the issue of patient understanding becomes especially challenging. Except in extraordinary circumstances (e.g., the patient described by Holmberg et al. 1996, already discussed), only patients with mild dementias should be considered for ECT. Patients in this group (sometimes defined as those with Mini-Mental State Examination scores between 20 and 24) (Folstein 1997; Folstein et al. 1975) can generally demonstrate adequate capacity for informed consent.

Electroconvulsive therapy also comes under close regulatory oversight. This may include the use of a mandated consent form, delineation of specific procedures to determine competence to consent, the need for a second psychiatric opinion that concurs with the administration of ECT, and special provisions for substituted consent. The administration of ECT to an incompetent patient may require a judge's order. Physicians should be familiar with the applicable local statutes or regulations.

Finally, the third element of consent involves the lack of coercion; patients should be informed that consent may be withdrawn at any time during the treatment series. Documentation of the consent process, with a copy for the patient, helps offer reassurance that information was provided and discussed. This also provides protection to the physician in rare cases in which undue influence or lack of adequate consent may be alleged.

Conducting Electroconvulsive Therapy

In the United States, ECT treatments are usually scheduled on a thrice-weekly basis (e.g., Monday, Wednesday, and Friday). A twice-weekly schedule may be recommended for patients with dementia; a longer recovery phase between treatments may lessen the cumulative nature of any cognitive side effects (Shapira et al. 1998). The disadvantage of this schedule is the longer time needed to administer an adequate number of treatments.

Electroconvulsive therapy should be administered by an adequately trained and privileged psychiatrist who is assisted by an anesthesiologist or experienced nurse anesthetist and an ECT nurse. Treatments are usually done in the morning, either in an ECT-dedicated area or in a hospital's day surgery or postanesthesia care unit. The patient must ingest nothing by mouth for at least 6–8 hours before the procedure; exceptions are made for cardiac or antireflux medications, which should be taken with a sip of water on the morning of the procedure. For patients with dementia, this may require written reminders (e.g., signs on faucets, cupboards, or the refrigerator) or one-on-one supervision.

Agitated patients may require pre-medication to lessen extreme agitation before the treatment. ECT can be easily coadministered with antipsychotic agents. Although several case reports suggest that trazodone may increase seizure duration (Lanes and Ravaris 1993), one of the authors (D.P.H.) has had good experience using it concomitantly with ECT. Benzodiazepines should be avoided because of their effects of raising the seizure threshold and contributing to daytime sedation, dizziness, and falls (a particular risk for elderly patients during a course of ECT). If a patient is receiving a benzodiazepine and ECT is given, the clinical efficacy of such a seizure is usually diminished even though the patient may have an adequate seizure duration.

The close monitoring of ECT with electrocardiography, pulse oximetry, blood pressure measurements, and electroencephalographic monitoring has dramatically increased its safety. The anesthesiologist should begin preoxygenation with 100% oxygen while the patient is conscious. After apnea is achieved, he or she hyperventilates the patient via bag and mask. Intravenous administration of the anesthetic, generally methohexital (a short-acting barbiturate), is followed by injection of succinylcholine to achieve neuromuscular blockade. For elderly patients who may have significant osteoporosis, the degree of muscular relaxation should be maximized; use of a nerve stimulator may help to confirm this.

When paralysis is adequate, the psychiatrist administers an electrical stimulus via electrodes placed either unilaterally (on the nondominant hemisphere) or bitemporally; the newer asymmetric bilateral position (Swartz and Evans 1996) is also an option. A therapeutic seizure often has a fairly characteristic electroencephalographic pattern; a minimum duration of 25 seconds peripherally and 40 seconds centrally is desirable. As the anesthetic wears off, the patient gradually awakens. Monitoring continues until the patient is fully alert and able to take sips of fluid, vital signs are stable, and oxygenation is adequate. Most patients return to their prior level of orientation within 60–120 minutes after the seizure.

Unilateral nondominant hemisphere electrode placement is associated with fewer cognitive side effects than bilateral placement. Most psychiatrists start with this modality in neurologically vulnerable patients. However, unilateral stimulation offers a less potent treatment effect, and some start with bilateral electrode placement for this reason. An effective unilateral stimulus must be delivered at suprathreshold doses. During the first session, the seizure threshold may be estimated, or it may be titrated according to the method described by Sackeim et al. (1993). If, after three or four treatments, unilateral electrode placement does not begin to yield clinical improvement, bilateral placement should be used thereafter. Similarly, if bilateral ECT is administered initially, careful monitoring of cognitive status is essential. If a decline occurs, a changeover to unilateral stimulus placement may be warranted.

Ongoing psychiatric care between treatments includes a careful assessment of both affective and cognitive functioning. In this way, the treating psychiatrist and the team can observe any subtle signs of improvement or worsening. A patient whose depressive symptoms are not improving and who exhibits stable cognitive functioning may do better with an increase in energy, a switch from unilateral to bilateral electrode placement, or both. Conversely, a patient who shows considerable improvement on a depression scale coincident with deterioration on the Mini-Mental State Examination may do best if switched from bilateral to unilateral placement and/or from thrice-weekly to once- or twice-weekly treatments. The acute series should continue until the patient's target symptoms are resolved or until no further improvement is observed between treatments.

Cardiac and Cognitive Side Effects and Their Management

The delivery of a convulsive stimulus causes significant hemodynamic changes. Initially, parasympathetic (vagal) tone increases; this may cause bradycardia or even several seconds of asystole. Seizure-induced sympathetic activation follows, with increased blood pressure and cardiac workload and decreased coronary-artery diastolic filling time. Postictally, vagal tone may again increase, and as the patient becomes conscious, sympathetic stimulation may again occur. Despite these rapid shifts, cardiovascular complications are rare in those without prior cardiac abnormalities; the type of preexisting disease (e.g., ischemia, rhythm disturbance) predicts ECT-related risk (Zielinski et al. 1993).

Anesthetic management can anticipate both physiological and pathological cardiac responses and protect patients with cardiovascular vulnerabilities. Pretreatment with an anticholinergic agent (e.g., atropine or glycopyrrolate) can counter vagal tone, but this benefit must be weighed against the risk of tachycardia. Subconvulsive stimuli may lead to excess vagal activity without a subsequent sympathetic response; use of the dose titration method may thereby increase the risk of bradycardia and asystole and tilt the scales toward pretreatment.

The routine use of prophylactic antihypertensive agents remains subject to debate. In patients without coronary artery disease, the hypertensive effects of ECT are transient and generally do not require treatment. Because both parasympathetic and sympathetic responses occur, the dangers of overshoot—especially bradycardia, hypotension, and decreased cerebral and cardiac perfusion—must be considered. For a patient whose myocardium cannot tolerate blood pressure rises, short-acting agents such as labetalol, esmolol, or sublingual nifedipine are favored.

The cognitive side effects of ECT are of three general types: acute postictal confusion, interictal disorientation and delirium, and amnesia. Acute postictal confusion occurs in the minutes or hours after an individual treatment. In a group of depressed, neurologically intact subjects, recovery of orientation took from 19.2 ± 10.5 minutes (high-dose right unilateral stimulus) to 40.0 ± 22.7 minutes (low-dose bitemporal stimulus) (Sobin et al. 1995). The time to reorientation is longer in older patients. A cumulative effect may also occur during a treatment series, particularly with thrice-weekly administration. As the patient returns to consciousness, it helps to reduce environmental noise and to have the treatment team member whom the patient knows best (i.e., the physician or the nurse) talk to the patient. We recommend speaking in simple, repetitive, declarative sentences, such as "You are waking up from your treatment. You may be confused; this is normal. You are in the hospital." Information acquired earlier in life will return faster than more recently acquired facts. Questions such as "Do you know where you are? You recognize me, don't you?" or nonspecific requests such as "Just relax" can increase agitation. In addition, because patients with dementia may be more prone to postictal confusion, the use of intravenous lorazepam after the seizure may be considered. Alternatively, a small amount of the anesthetic agent methohexital may be administered. This can keep the patient under sedation during the worst of the postictal confusion. Caution must be used to prevent excess respiratory depression.

Interictal disorientation and delirium may last beyond the several hours immediately after the treatment. They occur in a minority of patients and may be correlated with subcortical structural disease (discussed in Pritchett et al. 1994). If problematic behaviors result, treatments should be scheduled farther apart or a switch to unilateral electrode placement should be instituted.

Amnesia, both anterograde (i.e., difficulty retaining newly learned information) and retrograde (i.e., forgetting events before the treatment series) may also occur. Anterograde amnesia resolves relatively rapidly and is seldom seen for longer than 1 or 2 weeks after a treatment series. The duration of retrograde amnesia is more variable. Even after full recovery, some patients have little, if any, memory of events occurring during their hospital stay.

In their series, Sobin et al. (1995) investigated the duration of postictal disorientation and the extent of pre-ECT cognitive impairment as possible predictors of vulnerability to retrograde amnesia. At 1 week, among subjects treated with unilateral stimuli, postictal disorientation alone was predictive. For subjects receiving bilateral treatments, both variables were relevant. At 2 months, both factors had predictive value, independent of stimulus placement. Although it is unclear to what extent these finding are relevant for patients with dementia, the combination of significant cognitive impairment and prolonged postictal disorientation should promote caution in setting the treatment schedule.

Longitudinal studies of post-ECT cognitive measures often report unchanged or improved cognition when measured at periods from 6 months to 4 years after treatment (e.g., Stoudemire et al. 1995). Improved cognitive functioning is thought to be secondary to relief of the cognitive symptoms of depression. This can also be seen with the depressed patient with dementia, as demonstrated by some of the cases reviewed by Price and McAllister (1989). However, despite the lack of documented memory problems 6–9 months after ECT, subjective complaints may continue. In one series, 63% of subjects receiving bilateral ECT and 30% of those receiving unilateral stimuli (compared with 17% of those hospitalized without receiving ECT) believed that their ability to learn new material and recall familiar material was worse than before ECT (Squire and Chace 1975). It remains unknown whether the difference between objective and subjective measures might represent excess concern about memory dysfunction after ECT, inaccurate recall of pre-ECT functioning, or inadequacy of the testing instruments.

In terms of day-to-day management, patients and their families should be advised that the patient may lose information acquired over several months, including before, during, and after the treatment course. Important decisions should be delayed. For elderly patients with dementia, using cueing devices is even more important than usual, and adequate supervision should be provided until the convalescent phase ends.

Conclusions

Agitated behavior in patients with dementia may be associated with significant suffering, which presents a difficult challenge for caregivers and clinicians. Behavioral and pharmacological strategies are not always effective in reducing symptoms of agitation to a tolerable level. ECT has been used effectively to reduce agitation, especially in patients with dementia and depression, and should be considered for patients with severe, treatment-intolerant, or treatment-resistant illness. Cognitive side effects, when they occur, are usually time-limited and manageable, and modifications in technique can minimize side effects.

References

Abrams R: Electroconvulsive Therapy, 3rd Edition. New York, Oxford University Press, 1997

American Psychiatric Association: Diagnostic and Statistical Manual for Mental Disorders, 3rd Edition. Washington, DC, American Psychiatric Association, 1980

American Psychiatric Association: Diagnostic and Statistical Manual for Mental Disorders, 3rd Edition Revised. Washington, DC, American Psychiatric Association, 1987

American Psychiatric Association: The Practice of Electroconvulsive Therapy: Recommendations for Treatment, Training, and Privileging. Washington, DC, American Psychiatric Association, 1990

American Psychiatric Association: The Practice of Electroconvulsive Therapy: Recommendations for Treatment, Training, and Privileging, 2nd Edition. Washington, DC, American Psychiatric Association, 2001

Carlyle W, Killick L, Ancill R: ECT: an effective treatment in the screaming demented patient (letter). J Am Geriatr Soc 39:637, 1991

Coffey CE (ed): The Clinical Science of Electroconvulsive Therapy. Washington, DC, American Psychiatric Press, 1993

Folstein MF: Differential diagnosis of dementia. Psychiatr Clin North Am 20:45–57, 1997

Folstein MF, Folstein SE, McHugh PR: Mini-Mental State: a practical method for grading the cognitive state of patients for the clinician. J Psychiatr Res 12:189–198, 1975

Hay DP, Hay L, Grossberg GT: Electroconvulsive therapy for agitated dementia patients, in Treating Alzheimer's and Other Dementias: Clinical Application of Recent Research Advances. Edited by Bergener M, Finkel SI. New York, Springer, 1995, pp 415–426

Holmberg SK, Tariot PN, Challapalli R: Efficacy of ECT for agitation in dementia: a case report. Am J Geriatr Psychiatry 4:330–334, 1996

Lanes T, Ravaris C: Prolonged ECT seizure duration in a patient taking trazodone (letter). Am J Psychiatry 150:525, 1993

Nelson JP, Rosenberg DR: ECT treatment of demented elderly patients with major depression: a retrospective study of efficacy and safety. Convuls Ther 7:157–165, 1991

Price TR, McAllister TW: Safety and efficacy of ECT in depressed patients with dementia: a review of clinical experience. Convuls Ther 5:61–74, 1989

Pritchett JT, Kellner CH, Coffey CE: Electroconvulsive therapy in geriatric neuropsychiatry, in The American Psychiatric Press Textbook of Geriatric Neuropsychiatry. Edited by Coffey CE, Cummings JL. Washington, DC, American Psychiatric Press, 1994, pp 633–659

Sackeim HA, Prudic J, Devanand DP, et al: Effects of stimulus intensity and electrode placement on the efficacy and cognitive effects of electroconvulsive therapy. N Engl J Med 328:839–846, 1993

Schnur DB, Mukherjee S, Silver J, et al: Electroconvulsive therapy in the treatment of episodic aggressive dyscontrol in psychotic patients. Convuls Ther 5:353–361, 1989

Shapira B, Tubi N, Drexler H, et al: Cost and benefit in the choice of ECT schedule. Br J Psychiatry 172:44–48, 1998

Sobin C, Sackeim H, Prudic J, et al: Predictors of retrograde amnesia following ECT. Am J Psychiatry 152:995–1001, 1995

Squire LR, Chace PM: Memory functions six to nine months after electroconvulsive therapy. Arch Gen Psychiatry 32:1557–1564, 1975

Stoudemire A, Hill CD, Morris R, et al: Improvement in depression-related cognitive dysfunction following ECT. J Neuropsychiatry Clinical Neurosci 7:31–34, 1995

Swartz CM, Evans CM: Beyond bitemporal and right unilateral electrode placements. Psychiatr Ann 26:705–708, 1996

Zielinski RJ, Roose SP, Devand DP, et al: Cardiovascular complications of ECT in depressed patients with cardiac disease. Am J Psychiatry 150:904–909, 1993

Zwil AS, Pelchat RJ: ECT in the treatment of patients with neurological and somatic disease. International Journal of Psychiatry in Medicine 24:1–29, 1994

CHAPTER 15

Hormone Therapies

Mercedes M. Rodriguez, M.D.

Dementia is associated with a high prevalence of psychiatric symptoms and behavioral disturbances. These symptoms frequently present greater clinical challenges than cognitive deficits. Agitation, the most commonly reported behavioral symptom of dementia, refers to symptoms of disruptive behaviors, including inappropriate verbal outbursts, physical aggression, and nonpurposeful motor activity (Cohen-Mansfield 1986).

This spectrum of behavioral symptoms includes physical destructiveness, verbal disruptiveness, intrusiveness, sleep disturbances, impulsivity, and resistance to caregivers. Sexually inappropriate behavior and wandering can compromise the patient's safety. Agitation can occur in the context of depressive, anxious, and psychotic features. Whereas some studies show that physical aggression correlates highly with cognitive decline, others suggest that the severity of functional impairment is more predictive of disruptive behaviors (Devanand et al. 1992). Burns et al. (1990) reported an increase in severity of behavioral disturbances as cognitive decline progressed.

Therefore, the management of behavioral disturbances in patients with dementia may result in a significant improvement in quality of life of both caregivers and patients. Furthermore, unmodified behavioral disturbances in these patients are the leading causes of hospitalization and institutionalization (Ferris et al. 1987; Steele et al. 1990). The treatment of agitation in dementia includes behavioral, environmental, and milieu therapies as well as pharmacotherapy.

Various medications have been used, including antipsychotics, serotonergic agents, benzodiazepines, beta-blockers, anticonvulsants, lithium, buspirone, cholinesterase inhibitors, and hormones. In this chapter I present an overview of the role of hormones and their efficacy in decreasing aggressive behaviors in patients with dementia. Case reports help illustrate the type of patients who have been receiving hormones to control behavioral symptoms and the effect of hormones on these behaviors.

Link Between Agitation and Hormones

The deterioration of higher cortical functions in patients with dementia may decrease the patient's ability to appreciate the significance and meaning of various psychological, sociological, and environmental factors that normally inhibit aggressive behaviors in persons without dementia. Reproductive hormones can mediate the expression of aggression (Rodriguez and Grossberg 1998). The mechanism of action of androgens, estrogens, and their metabolites on human behavior is not clear. It is likely to have multiple direct and indirect effects on thought, cognition, and behavior (Cohen 1988; MacLean 1985).

Studies conducted in animals suggest that physical aggression in men may be linked to testosterone and/or its metabolites and that it may be reduced with bilateral orchiectomy or the administration of estrogen and/or its metabolites (Barfield 1984; Beeman 1947; Bouissou 1983; Floody and Pfaff 1974; Moyers 1974). However, these studies have not addressed the issue of efficacy. These studies have also not correlated procedure or blood estrogen levels to the temporal course of behavioral response. Gonadal hormones have been shown to considerably influence brain receptors (McEwen 1987). There is also mostly indirect evidence that they are involved in modulation of behavior and mood in humans (McEwen 1987). This involvement is through hormonal interaction with neurotransmitters and other neuromodulators. There is a body of data indicating that estrogen and progesterone influence synthesis, metabolism, uptake, and turnover as well as receptor sites and mechanisms of serotonin, among other neurotransmitters (Rovner et al. 1986).

A number of steroids have been synthesized with progestinal and antiandrogenic properties. These substances were developed originally as oral contraceptives and for menstrual and pregnancy disorders. However, they have found wider applications in disturbances of behavior (e.g., agitation, aberrant sexual behavior, inappropriate behavior) (Rovner et al. 1986). The three most familiar of this class of drugs are medroxyprogesterone acetate (MPA; Provera, Depo-Provera), cyproterone acetate (CPA; Androcur), and conjugated equine estrogens (CEE). These hormones are available in Western Europe and the United Kingdom. In the United States and Canada, only MPA and CEE are being used to suppress deviant behavior. Since 1966, MPA has been used to treat sexual offenders of various types (Kreutz and Rose 1972), and most investigators observed a significant decrease in sexual tension, fantasies, and preoccupations and masturbation.

Review of Studies

Studies in Men

Human studies indicate that testosterone increases aggression in men. Studies in prisoners have found that violent male offenders show substantially higher plasma testosterone levels than less violent offenders (Kreutz and Rose 1972). Men are most often convicted of aggressive crimes, and there is increased energy expenditure in the rough-and-tumble play of boys (Moyers 1974) and in children with congenital adrenogenital syndrome (Ehrhardt and Baker 1974). Anabolic androgenic steroid use in athletes also has been associated with increased aggression (Christiansen and Knussman 1987; Conacher and Workman 1989). In contrast, the removal of the predominant source of testosterone or the administration of estrogen compounds has resulted in reduced aggressiveness and sexually offensive behavior in some men (Bell 1978; Moyers 1974).

Gagne (1981) used MPA to treat 48 men who had long histories of deviant sexual behavior (e.g., pedophilia, exhibitionism, transvestism). In the first 2 weeks, patients received MPA 200 mg intramuscularly two to three times a week. During the next 4 weeks, they received 200 mg once or twice a week, depending on the clinical response. Then the MPA continued to be tapered until patients received 100 mg/week. Treatment was monitored by measuring testosterone levels every 2 weeks for the first month and then monthly afterwards. Within 3 weeks, 40 of 48 patients responded positively, with diminished sexual fantasies and arousal and decreased desire for sexual behavior (e.g., masturbation, ejaculation). These improvements were maintained after treating patients for 12 months. In most cases, testosterone levels fell to less than half of their initial values after only four injections of MPA. All patients had improvement in psychosexual functioning in the first 2 months. Adverse effects consisted of fatigue, weight gain, insomnia, headaches, and nausea.

In another study, Money (1970) treated 10 patients who had paraphilias. He administered MPA 200 mg intramuscularly once a week. Results included reduced frequency of erotic imagery as well as reduced frequency of erections and masturbation. Some men stopped the offensive behavior entirely for 2 years. After treatment, several patients stopped deviant behavior entirely, reporting relief from pressure to act on troublesome sexual urges while still maintaining the capacity for intercourse. Presumably, the decreased frequency of erotic thoughts comes about, at least in part, as a consequence of lowered levels of testosterone.

In another study (Berlin and Meinecke 1981), 20 men with histories of chronically recurrent paraphiliac behavior were given MPA for varying lengths of time. In this study, only 3 patients showed recurrences of sexually deviant behavior while taking the medication; in one such case, relapse was clearly related to alcohol abuse. The relapse rate jumped dramatically when patients discontinued MPA against medical advice. Eleven patients discontinued the drug against medical advice, and 10 relapsed. The conclusions of this study suggest that patients appear to do well in response to antiandrogenic medication as long as they continue taking it. They seem to do less well if they have been noncompliant about taking the medication or if they have comorbid use of alcohol or drugs. Similar correlations occurred in volunteer male samples divided according to the presence or absence of aggression when drinking alcohol or playing a competitive sport (Steele et al. 1990).

The relationship between testosterone and aggression in men with dementia has not been systematically investigated, but case studies have reported the efficacy of estrogen treatment for aggression in two men with dementia and in one case of traumatic brain injury (Kyomen et al. 1997).

Arnold (1993) reported on a patient who, after traumatic brain injury with chronic, severe agitation refractory to treatment, responded to a low-dose trial of estrogen (0.625–1.25 mg/day). This patient had a marked decrease of agitated behavior by the end of the first week and a near total resolution of aggressive behavior after the first week of treatment. At 4 months' follow-up, the patient revealed sustained improvement.

In a study by Orengo et al. (1997), an association between aggressive behavior and high levels of plasma testosterone was noted. In 13 subjects (8 white, 5 black; mean age 76.5 years; mean Mini-Mental State Examination [MMSE] score 10.1; mean plasma testosterone level 8.9 pg/mL [range 2.1–19.1]), the testosterone level was found to be positively associated with a decrease in agitation (measured by the Overt Aggression Scale [Ray et al. 1992] and the Cohen-Mansfield Agitation Scale). Because of the small sample size (i.e., 13 subjects), they did not investigate the correlation between aggression and testosterone in subgroups of patients with different types of dementia.

Amadeo (1996) reported on three patients with probable dementia of the Alzheimer type (DAT) who manifested an aggressive syndrome and motor disturbances, including agitation, pacing, and restlessness. The patients were treated successfully with the antiandrogenic agents MPA acetate and luprolide acetate. Within 4 weeks of the start of the MPA, verbal and physical aggressivity ceased and activity disturbances such as agitation, pacing, and restlessness were markedly reduced. One patient also manifested marked disinhibited and disruptive sexual behavior; after treatment, that behavior also ceased. The major adverse effects reported in this study were sleepiness, mild diabetes, increased appetite, hair loss, hot and cold flashes, depression, and reduced ejaculation.

Kyomen et al. (1991) conducted a similar study using estrogen instead of MPA for the reduction of physically aggressive behavior in two men with severe DAT. In both cases, estrogen reduced the number of incidents of physical aggression but not verbal aggression. The side effects of estrogen therapy in men include fluid retention, hypophosphatemia, gynecomastia, and decreased libido, and there are conflicting reports about the cardiovascular benefits or risks of estrogen therapy (Kyomen et al. 1997). The use of small doses of estrogen in men is thought to be associated with a low side-effect profile. The patients studied experienced no adverse effects from the estrogen.

Cooper (1986) studied four institutionalized men, one of whom had mild to moderate dementia and three of whom had moderate dementia. These patients manifested disruptive sexual behavior, including public masturbation and attempts to molest female patients, and could not be managed by other means. They received a therapeutic trial of 300 mg/week of MPA for 1 year and were followed for 1 additional year. Sexual activities were recorded before, during, and after the study. Serum testosterone, luteinizing hormone, and prolactin were measured regularly. By 2 weeks after initiation of MPA therapy, the sexual acting-out stopped; this was associated with a 90% and a 60% decline, respectively, of serum testosterone and luteinizing hormone. When MPA was stopped, testosterone and luteinizing hormone returned to pretrial levels in all four men. There were no adverse effects, and laboratory values remained within normal limits. It was concluded from this small study that MPA was successful in suppressing unacceptable sexual behavior and that it was associated with marked reduction in testosterone levels.

Medroxyprogesterone acetate has also been used effectively as treatment in studies of patients with schizophrenia who manifested sexual delusions and compulsive masturbation; in a small number of people with mental retardation; and in a few cases of sexually disinhibited, cognitively intact elderly men (Cooper 1986; Hoffet 1968). One report by Potocnik (1992) described the successful treatment with CPA of hypersexuality in a patient with dementia due to AIDS.

All of the studies described thus far involved the treatment of agitation in men and noted minimal adverse adverse effects, making hormones an attractive alternative in the treatment of agitation.

Studies in Women

Estrogen, progesterone, and androgen may have a significant effect on the restoration of libido in women. Perloff (1949) reported that estrogen therapy is effective in increasing sexual drive in postmenopausal women. These reports are more than two decades old and are based on unstructured clinical interviews. Bakke (1983) reported a double-blind, placebo-controlled study that evaluated hormone replacement therapy in postmenopausal women. His findings suggested a clear-cut effect on libido. The sample of 27 women had blind trials with all three agents consecutively.

The endocrine contribution to women's sexual behavior is complex and poorly understood despite the coincidence of reports of sexual dysfunction and the dramatic decline in ovarian hormone levels at menopause (Rovner et al. 1986). Although a decrease in sexual activity in a significant percentage of menopausal women is well established, these data are still inadequate to ascribe reported decreases to specific hormonal changes (McCoy and Davidson 1985).

Several studies have examined the effect of hormones on behavior in women. Dennerstein et al. (1979) and Sherwin and Gelfand (1987) have published the results of controlled, double-blind studies of hormone replacement therapy in subjects who had undergone surgical menopause (i.e., hysterectomy and oophorectomy). These studies suggest a positive effect between synthetic steroids and sexuality (increased libido, masturbation, and orgasm), leaving doubt as to whether the effects were physiological or pharmacological.

In a double-blind, placebo-controlled clinical trial, Kyomen et al. (1997) evaluated the efficacy of estrogens in decreasing aggressive behaviors in elderly long-term care residents with severe dementia. Of 13 patients studied, 12 were women and 1 was a man. Placebo or conjugated estrogen was given in doses of 0.625 mg during the first week, 1.25 mg the second week, 1.875 mg the third week, and 2.5 mg the fourth week, with minimal adverse effects. This study showed a decrease in the frequency of physically aggressive behaviors. Cognitive abilities also showed a trend toward improvement. The patients studied experienced no adverse effects from the estrogen.

Ethical and Medicolegal Issues

There may be ethical and medicolegal issues regarding the use of hormones to treat agitation or sexually deviant behavior. A detailed discussion is presented in Chapter 16. If a decision is made to use hormones to treat behavior in a patient with dementia and the patient is competent, informed consent needs to be obtained in writing. Each patient must be assessed carefully on an individual basis, and the physician, patient, and family should attempt to balance as best they can the rights and needs of the patient against those of society. If the patient lacks the capacity to make decisions because of the severity of the dementia or the presence of psychosis, consent must be obtained from the legal guardian.

Case Vignette

The following case illustrates the type of patient who may benefit from hormone therapy.

> Mr. A, an 82-year-old man with a diagnosis of probable DAT with behavioral disturbances, as defined by National Institute of Neurological and Communicative Disorders and Stroke and the Alzheimer's Disease and Related Disorders Associations (NINCDS-ADRDA) criteria, was admitted to an inpatient geriatric psychiatry unit for management of agitation. His agitated behavior consisted of kicking and spitting at the nursing staff, banging and shaking, wandering in the ward and trying to leave the nursing home by opening all the doors, yelling constantly, not sleeping at night, throwing and spitting his food when fed, hitting staff members when they attempted to shower him, and masturbating in the halls of the nursing home.
>
> The patient's behavioral disturbances had been treated previously using multiple combinations of medications, among them benzodiazepines (lorazepam, clonazepam), anticonvulsants (valproic acid, carbamazepine, gabapentin), antidepressants (paroxetine, sertraline, trazodone), antipsychotics (haloperidol, risperidone) and beta-blockers (propanolol), without adequate response. His past medical history was significant for a diagnosis of prostatic hypertrophy. On admission, a complete physical examination was performed, which was unremarkable except for a mildly dry oral mucosa. The neurological examination was unremarkable. A computed tomography scan of the head revealed generalized cerebral atrophy. Blood work was within normal range. A urinalysis did reveal a urinary tract infection, which was treated with antibiotics. Vital

signs were stable. The mental status examination revealed an 82-year-old white man who looked his stated age, who was difficult to redirect, who appeared thin, and who had psychomotor agitation. He was pacing constantly, without involuntary movements or parkinsonian movements, but with anxious mood and affect. He denied perceptual disturbances. He had no suicidal ideas or plans, and his sensorium was clear. Folstein MMSE results were 10. In the functional assessment, the patient showed impairment in his activities of daily living (e.g., bathing, shaving, dressing) and instrumental activities of daily living (e.g., using the telephone, doing finances).

After review of the pros and cons of hormone treatment with the patient's family and legal guardian (the patient's wife), it was decided to prescribe MPA. Informed consent was obtained, and the patient was started on intramuscular MPA 150 mg/week for 2 weeks. This was increased to 200 mg/week thereafter. The patient was discharged from the hospital after obtaining good control of agitation symptoms. His pretreatment testosterone levels were 567 ng/100 mL. After treatment, repeated monthly determinations averaged 150 ng/mL (the objective is to have levels lower than 250 ng/100 mL).

After 2 months of treatment with MPA, treatment effects reported by the nursing home staff and by the family were as follows:

- The patient's agitation was controlled.
- The patient's sleep was improved, with occasional awakening at night.
- The patient exhibited appetite with weight gain.
- The patient was able to be managed in the nursing home, with a decreasing number of visits to the emergency room and admissions to the hospital.

Conclusions

Behavioral disturbances in patients with dementia greatly increase patient morbidity as well as the stress, strain, and burden on patients' family and professional caregivers. A great deal of work needs to be done to further elucidate the neurochemical mechanisms that underlie these syndromes. However, there are behavioral, psychosocial, environmental, and pharmacological interventions now available to help control the manifestations of symptoms associated with dementia. Pharmacologically, there is little doubt that hormones are preferable to other currently available medications because of their benign side effect profile and efficacy. They may now be considered equal to the other psychotropic medications. They should be begun at low doses and gradually titrated upward while closely monitoring for adverse effects, including increasing agitation or confusion.

At present, it is not known how long hormones need to be taken or can safely be taken. A reasonable compromise suggested by the literature is to prescribe these medications at optimal levels for approximately 2 years. Then the patient should be reevaluated and a decision may be made regarding the possibility of tapering the dose or stopping it completely. If this action is taken, the patient should be closely monitored, and any signs of relapse should result in immediate reinstitution of the drug at former therapeutic levels. However, more studies are needed to define more precisely the long-term behavioral and biological effects of these agents and their limitations.

References

Amadeo M: Antiandrogen treatment of aggressivity in men suffering from dementia. J Geriatr Psychiatry Neurol 9:142–45, 1996

Arnold SE: Estrogen for refractory aggression after traumatic brain injury. Am J Psychiatry 150:1564–1565, 1993

Barfield RJ: Reproductive hormones and aggressive behavior. Prog Clin Biol Res 169:105–134, 1984

Beeman EA: The effect of male hormone on aggressive behavior in mice. Physiological Zoology 20:373–405, 1947

Bell R: Hormone influences on human aggression. Ir J Med Sci 147(suppl):5–9, 1978

Berlin FS, Meinecke CG: Treatment of sex offenders with antiandrogenic medication: conceptualization, review of treatment modalities, and preliminary findings. Am J Psychiatry 138:601–607, 1981

Bakke L: A double-blind study of progestin–estrogen combination in the management of the menopause. Pacific Medical Surgical May–June 1983, p 200

Bouissou M: Androgens, aggressive behavior and social relationships in higher mammals. Horm Res 18:43–61, 1983

Burns A, Jacoby R, Levy R: Psychiatric phenomenon in Alzheimer's disease, IV: disorders of behavior. Br J Psychiatry 157:86–94, 1990

Christiansen K, Knussman R: Androgen levels and components of aggressive men. Horm Behav 21:170–180, 1987

Cohen GD: The Brain in Human Aging. New York, Springer, 1988

Cohen-Mansfield J: Agitated behaviors in the elderly, II: preliminary results in the cognitively deteriorated. J Am Geriatr Soc 34:722–727, 1986

Conacher GN, Workman DG: Violent crime possibly associated with anabolic steroid use (letter). Am J Psychiatry 146:679, 1989

Cooper AJ: Progestogens in the treatment of male sexual offenders: a review. Can J Psychiatry 31:73–79, 1986

Dennerstein L, Burrows GD, Hyman GJ, et al: Hormone therapy and affect. Maturitas 1:247–59, 1979

Devanand DP, Brockington CD, Moody BJ, et al: Behavioral syndromes in Alzheimer's disease. Int Psychogeriatr 4:161–184, 1992

Ehrhardt AA, Baker SW: Fetal androgens, human central nervous system differentiation, and behavior sex differences, in Sex Differences in Behavior. Edited by Friedman RC, Richardt RM, Van de Wiele RL. New York, Wiley, 1974, pp 33–51

Ferris SH, Steinberg G, Shulman E, et al: Institutionalization of Alzheimer's disease patients, reducing precipitating factors through family counseling. Home Health Care Serv Q 8:23–51, 1987

Floody OR, Pfaff DW: Steroid hormones and aggressive behavior: approaches to the study of hormone-sensitive brain mechanisms for behavior. Res Publ Assoc Res Nerv Ment Dis 52:149–185, 1974

Gagne P: Treatment of sex offenders with medroxyprogesterone acetate. Am J Psychiatry 138:644–646, 1981

Hoffet H: The treatment of sexual delinquents and psychiatric hospital patients with the testosterone blocker cyproterone acetate (SH 714). Praxis 577:221–230, 1968

Kreutz LE, Rose RM: Assessment of aggressive behavior and plasma testosterone in a young criminal population. Psychosom Med 34:321–332, 1972

Kyomen HH, Nobel KW, Wei JY: The use of estrogen to decrease aggressive physical behavior in elderly men with dementia. J Am Geriatr Soc 39:1110–1112, 1991

Kyomen HH, Satlin A, Wei JY, et al: Estrogen therapy decreases physically aggressive behaviors in elderly long-term care facility dementia patients: results from a double blind, placebo-controlled clinical trial. J Neuropsychiatry Clin Neurosci 9:174, 1997

MacLean PD: Evolutionary psychiatry and the triune brain. Psychol Med 15:219–221, 1985

McCoy N, Davidson JM: A longitudinal study of the effects of menopause on sexuality. Maturitas 7:203–210, 1985

McEwen B: Gonadal and adrenal steroids and the brain: implications for depression, in Hormones and Depression. Edited by Halbreich U. New York, Raven, 1987, pp 239–251

Money J: Use of an androgen-depleting hormone in the treatment of male sex offenders. Journal of Sex Research 6:165–172, 1970

Moyers KE: Sex differences in aggression, in Sex Differences in Behavior. Edited by Friedman RC, Richardt RM, Van de Wiele RL. New York, Wiley, 1974, pp 335–372

Orengo CA, Kunik ME, Ghusn H, et al: Correlation of testosterone with aggression in demented elderly men. J Nerv Ment Dis 185:349–351, 1997

Perloff H: Role of the hormones in human sexuality. Psychosom Med 11:333–372, 1949

Potocnik F: Successful treatment of hypersexuality in AIDS dementia with cyproterone acetate. S Afr Med J 18:433–434, 1992

Ray WA, Taylor JA, Lichtenstein MJ, et al: The Nursing Home Behavior Problem Scale. J Gerontol 47:M9–M16, 1992

Rodriguez MM, Grossberg GT: Estrogen as a psychotherapeutic agent. Clin Geriatr Med 14:177–190, 1998

Rovner BW, Kafonek S, Filipp L, et al: Prevalence of mental illness in a community nursing home. Am J Psychiatry 143:1446–1449, 1986

Sherwin BB, Gelfand MM: The role of androgen in the maintenance of sexual functioning in oophorectomized women. Psychosom Med 49:397–409, 1987

Steele C, Rovner B, Chasse A, et al: Psychiatric symptoms and nursing home placement with Alzheimer's disease. Am J Psychiatry 147:1049–1051, 1990

CHAPTER 16

Legal and Ethical Issues

Barbara J. Gilchrist, J.D., Ph.D.

Alice was diagnosed with dementia, probably of the Alzheimer's type, several years ago. She was able to remain in her own home with her husband with the help of in-home aides until recently, when her husband fell and broke his hip. Alice's adult children were not able to provide the care and supervision she requires, so the family made the very difficult decision to place Alice in a nursing home. Shortly after this move, Alice began physically striking out at the nursing home attendants and shouting at other residents, sometimes using curse words. On several occasions, she refused to take her medications, which include a drug to control her hypertension, and she has been wandering much more than when she was in her own home.

The scenario above presents very difficult legal and ethical issues for medical and nursing home professionals as well as family members. Every patient, whatever his or her particular diagnosis, prognosis, mental or physical limitations, or family structure, has the same array of legal rights. These rights include autonomy, informed consent, refusal of treatment, freedom from confinement, and the naming of a proxy or surrogate for decision-making purposes. None of these rights, however, is absolute. Each individual right must be balanced against broader social rights such as the right of others not to be harmed and sometimes conflicting individual rights such as the right to receive adequate and appropriate treatment. Alice's cognitive limitations reduced her ability to control her life and precipitated the nursing home placement. And, of course, after Alice was moved into a nursing home, her autonomy was constrained to some degree. As recognized by Hayley et al. (1996), "moving from a familiar setting of former independence to the nursing home confirms and adds a new dimension to the loss of autonomy and self-determination."

Any discussion of the rights of patients must be set in a specific context because it is in the application of these rights that conflict may arise. An agitated patient with dementia adds the complication of physical and psychological dependence (Kitwood 1998), which raises the question of whether a substitute decision maker is needed.

For purposes of this discussion, it is assumed that Alice has been diagnosed with dementia but has not been adjudicated as legally incompetent or incapacitated. She is a patient with midstage dementia who is in need of behavioral management interventions (Kovach 1996). Furthermore, it is assumed that Alice's behavior is impeding the care providers in their efforts to fulfill their medical responsibilities to her and that there is some risk of physical harm to Alice or others. What follows is a description of the legal principles that must be taken into account to balance the preservation of Alice's rights with the management of her treatment.

Autonomy

Autonomy is the guiding principle in medical ethics and is closely tied to legal concepts of privacy and informed consent. In a nursing home environment, however, autonomy may be lost in the day-to-day delivery of care to residents. Federal and state regulations require nursing homes to have established policies and procedures to ensure quality and safety, sometimes at the cost of individual attention (Hayley et al. 1996). This loss is exacerbated for patients with dementia (Kitwood 1998), whose cognitive limitations remove them even further from the "opportunit[y] to enter into meaningful decisions" (Smith 1996, p. 36).

With some effort, nursing homes can make allowances for individual autonomy, "[w]hether it is the right to have visitors or the right to privacy in using the bathroom when feasible or the right to decide whether to undergo a medical test or procedure" (Hayley et al. 1996, p. 250). At the same time, autonomy should not become an excuse for abandoning a resistant patient whose resistance may be symptomatic of an underlying illness (Smith 1996).

Competency

Every adult is legally presumed to be competent until there has been a judicial determination to the contrary. Every competent adult, with few exceptions, is allowed to determine the course of his or her medical treatment, even when the patient refuses life-saving treatment (Brown 1997). A diagnosis of dementia or any other form of mental illness does not automatically mean that the individual is also incompetent, but when a patient with dementia begins to exhibit signs of agitation and some change in treatment or intervention is needed, three separate and distinct questions must be asked:

1. Does this individual retain some capacity to make a medical decision?
2. Is this individual a danger to him- or herself or others?
3. What is the least restrictive environment in which necessary treatment may be provided?

The answers to these questions determine the action that must be taken.

Decisional Capacity

The standards for decisional capacity in a medical context are not always the same as the criteria a court would apply in determining competency or legal capacity (Smith 1996). Legal incapacity is a much broader and less refined concept, and it is absolute. A person is either competent or incompetent for all purposes. Therefore, some patients who might be found legally incompetent by a court do, in fact, have the ability, from a medical perspective, to understand the consequences of accepting or foregoing a particular treatment. "[L]imited decision-making capacity does not mean that [the patient is] completely unable to make decisions…For instance, the level of understanding required for consent to draw blood is considerably less than that required for elective surgery because of the higher relative risk" (Hayley et al. 1996, p. 252).

A difficult situation occurs when a patient who has some level of decisional capacity is, in the opinion of the physician, making a bad choice, perhaps for reasons that are not rational. This is especially troubling when a patient refuses medication that would be expected to reduce the level of agitation or remove the underlying cause of the agitation. Kapp (1998) warns, however, against restricting patient choice out of fear of liability on the part of providers or family members if a patient with questionable capacity makes a bad choice.

If, after careful review of clinical alternatives, the physician believes that the patient cannot understand the information and options being provided and cannot make a rational decision (Kapp 1998), it may be time for a health care proxy to step in, or there may need to be a petition filed with the appropriate court for a determination of incapacity and the appointment of a guardian.

Danger to Self or Others and Involuntary Hospitalization

If a patient with some level of decisional capacity is physically aggressive or is behaving in ways that place him or her at risk of serious physical harm, the physician must consider involuntary hospitalization if other, less restrictive alternatives will not adequately protect the patient or others (Kapp 1992). State procedures and requirements for involuntary commitment vary, but they typically allow for short-term emergency confinement followed by a judicial procedure to determine if the patient will continue to be hospitalized on an involuntary basis and for what period of time. In any such court proceeding, there must be "clear and convincing evidence" that, at a minimum, the patient is mentally ill and is dangerous to self or others (Addington v. Texas 1979). If involuntary hospitalization is ordered by a court, the order is subject to periodic review and will be terminated when the patient's circumstances no longer meet the statutory requirements.

It is important to recognize that a court order allowing for involuntary hospitalization does not mean that the individual has been determined to be legally incompetent nor has the patient lost the right to refuse treatment (Kapp 1992). In the context of an agitated dementia patient, involuntary hospitalization, when necessary, may need to be coupled with a guardianship for treatment to proceed.

Prior Directive

Most, if not all, states have legislation that recognizes the right of a competent adult to identify a surrogate or proxy to make health care decisions in the event of incapacity. In addition, the federal Patient Self Determination Act requires hospitals, nursing homes, and certain other medical facilities receiving federal funds to provide residents with information about these rights under state law. Specifically, facilities must provide "written information to each…individual concerning an individual's rights under state law…to make decisions concerning…the right to formulate advance directives" (42 USCA §1395cc[f][1][A] [Supp 2001]).

Written documents identifying a substitute decision maker may be called *advance medical directives, health care powers of attorney,* or other similar names, depending on the state statute and local practice. They sometimes also include directions as to the patient's wishes at the very end of life.

If Alice, for example, has named her husband or one of her children (or anyone else of her choosing) as her surrogate in a written document, the surrogate is authorized to make whatever medical decisions may arise after it has been medically documented that Alice can no longer competently do this for herself. Health care providers should recognize the authority of the proxy, even in the face of disagreement from the patient or other family members.

Alice's decisional capacity may fluctuate, and the proxy's authority should be adjusted accordingly. In other words, after a proxy has been appropriately allowed to step in and begin to give the health care provider direction, it does not mean that the patient has permanently lost the right to control his or her treatment. Rather, there should be an ongoing dynamic process of evaluating the patient's ability to participate in the decision-making process. For example, Alice's proxy may appropriately consent to a course of treatment that results in a reduction in agitated behaviors and an increase in Alice's ability to rationally understand and respond to her treatment needs. At that point, at least some, if not all, of the decision making should shift back to Alice. As noted previously, Alice may be able to participate in making simpler medical decisions while her surrogate provides direction when the question requires more complex reasoning abilities.

Before allowing a substitute decision maker to give direction in medical decisions, a copy of the authorizing document should be placed in the patient's records and the document should be carefully reviewed to determine whether there are any limitations on the authority granted.

In the absence of a written prior directive, a process called *substituted judgment* is often followed to determine the care that will be provided for a patient who, although not adjudicated as incapacitated, is actually unable to give meaningful direction (Brock 1996). This means that the care provider consults with those persons close to the patient who have knowledge of what the patient would or would not want done. This process is not recognized in all states (notably New York and Missouri) and may not be appropriate at all for an agitated patient with dementia who is verbally and physically resistant. It may be necessary for someone to become Alice's guardian.

Guardianship

The requirements for establishing a guardianship (or conservatorship) are also set by state law and vary from one state to another. In all cases, however, a petition must be filed with the court (typically probate or family court) and a hearing held. Evidence of the patient's need for a guardian will be presented, and the court will determine whether the individual meets the state statutory definition of incompetency or incapacity and will appoint someone as the guardian if the standard has been met. The Uniform Probate Code, as an example, defines an "incapacitated person" as

> an individual who, for reasons other than being a minor, is unable to receive and evaluate information or make or communicate decisions to such an extent that the individual lacks the ability to meet essential requirements for physical health, safety, or self-care, even with appropriate technological assistance. (UPC, Article V, Part 1 §5–102[4] [1998])

After a patient has been determined to be legally incompetent, he or she loses all civil rights, including the right to consent to or refuse treatment. The authority over (and responsibility for) all of these rights now resides with the guardian. However, there may be limitations on the guardian's authority to consent to involuntary hospitalization as well as authority to terminate certain types of life-supporting treatment without court permission.

Physicians and other health care providers have a dual role in the guardianship process. First, they may identify for the family the patient who is in need of a guardian. Secondly, after a guardianship proceeding has been initiated, a medical evaluation is required by the court, and the medical expert provides this information, either in written form or by testifying at a hearing (Kapp 1992).

Least Restrictive Alternative

The legal principle of *least restrictive alternative* grew out of a recognition that, in the context of mentally ill patients, treatment should be delivered in an environment that least restricts the patient's civil rights. This concept encompasses both the general setting in which care is delivered and the specific limitations placed on an individual patient (Ziegenfuss 1983). As stated by Ziegenfuss (1983), "[t]he process by which this right is protected is a continuous and ongoing exploration of alternatives." Similar principles are applied in a guardianship context as well. For example, the Uniform Probate Code admonishes the court, in its appointment of a guardian, "to encourage the development of maximum self-reliance and independence of the incapacitated person and make appointive and other orders only to the extent necessitated by the incapacitated person's mental and adaptive limitations" (UPC, Article V. Part 1, §5-306 [1998]).

Freedom From Restraints

Federal law requires nursing homes to "protect and promote the rights of each resident," including:

> The right to be free from physical or mental abuse, corporal punishment, involuntary seclusion, and any physical or chemical restraints imposed for purposes of discipline or convenience and not required to treat the resident's medical symptoms. Restraints may only be imposed
> (I) to ensure the physical safety of the resident or other residents, and
> (II) only upon the written order of a physician that specifies the duration and circumstances under which the restraints are to be used (except in emergency circumstances...until such an order could reasonably be obtained). (42 USCA §1396r[c][1][A][ii] [Supp 2001])

A common reason given for the use of physical restraints is to prevent falls, but a recent study of the relationship between restraint reduction and the rate of falls concludes that removing physical restraints does not increase falls or related injuries in nursing home residents (Capezuti et al. 1998). Other empirical research has shown that, rather than reducing injury, restraints increase the risk of death by strangulation, increase agitation, and exacerbate conditions caused by immobility (Johnson 1990; Lach 1993).

Federal law further restricts the use of chemical restraints by requiring a written plan of treatment "designed to eliminate or modify the symptoms for which the drugs are prescribed " (42 USCA §1396r[D] [1992]). Studies cited by Meyers and Cahenzli (1993) indicate that psychotropic drugs are widely prescribed for nursing home residents, especially to treat agitation. As stated by these authors, "[t]he central question is whether psychotropics are prescribed for a putative therapeutic activity or as a means of managing unacceptable behavior by sedation. Are medications administered to chemically restrain and thereby control nursing home residents or to treat disorders?"

The controversy over which drugs to prescribe and when to prescribe them has not been resolved. Meyers and Cahenzli (1993) recommend that until sufficient empirical research has been completed, health care providers refer to the clinical studies that are available and practice "within regulatory guidelines."

Conclusions

The scenario described at the beginning of this chapter presents a set of difficult circumstances for family, physicians, and other care providers, made all the more difficult by the dependence of the person suffering from dementia. The answer to what is to happen with Alice lies in a process of balancing her ability to exercise her autonomy with her need for care. Ideally, a graduated approach to resolving the current difficulties will be used, beginning with her family, physician, and the care providers at the nursing home in an effort to find ways to help Alice feel more comfortable with the nursing home setting. This may serve to reduce the anxiety caused by the move. Perhaps a change in medication is warranted. If Alice is unwilling or unable to consent, her surrogate may need to step in. If Alice has not named a surrogate in a prior directive, the family and physician will have to decide whether a guardianship is now necessary. It is unlikely that involuntary hospitalization would be appropriate as long as Alice's behavior does not escalate to a point where it cannot be managed in the nursing home.

Finding the balance between autonomy and beneficence in the treatment of an agitated patient with dementia is a difficult and dynamic process. As Alice's limitations increase over time, her ability to control her care will diminish. Allowing her participation for as long as possible is the challenge.

References

Addington v Texas, 441 U.S. 418 (1979)

Brock D: What is the moral authority of family members to act as surrogates of incompetent patients? Milbank Q 74:599–618, 1996

In re Brown, 294 Ill. App. 3d 159, 689 N.E. 2d 397, 228 Ill. Dec. 525 (1997)

Capezuti E, Strumpf NE, Evans LK, et al: The relationship between physical restraint removal and falls and injuries among nursing home residents. Journals of Gerontology, Series A 53:M47–M52, 1998

Hayley DC, Cassel CK, Snyder l, et al: Ethical and legal issues in nursing home care. Arch Intern Med 156:249–256, 1996

Johnson S: The fear of liability and the use of restraints in nursing homes. Law, Medicine and Health Care 18:263–273, 1990

Kapp MB: Geriatrics and the Law: Patient Rights and Professional Responsibilities, 2nd Edition. New York, Springer, 1992

Kapp MB: Persons with dementia as "liability magnets": ethical implications. J Clin Ethics 9:66–70, 1998

Kitwood T: Toward a theory of dementia care: ethics and interaction. J Clin Ethics 9:23–34, 1998

Kovach CR: Alzheimer's disease: long-term care issues. Issues in Law and Medicine 12:47–56, 1996

Lach HW: Use of Physical Restraints and Options in Problem Behaviors in Long-Term Care: Recognition, Diagnosis, and Treatment. Edited by Szwabo PA, Grossberg GT. New York, Springer, 1993, pp 176–187

Meyers BS, Cahenzli CT: Psychotropics in the extended care facility, in Long-Term Care: Recognition, Diagnosis, and Treatment. Edited by Szwabo PA, Grossberg GT. New York, Springer, 1993, pp 81–93

Smith GP: Legal and Healthcare Ethics for the Elderly. Washington, DC, Taylor and Francis, 1996

Ziegenfuss JT: Patient's Rights and Professional Practice. New York, Van Nostrand Reinhold, 1983

Index

*Page numbers printed in **boldface** type refer to tables and figures.*

231